Psychoanalysis and Severe Disorders in Young Children

W0234892

Psychoanalysis and Severe Disorders in Young Children presents case material and resources for professionals working with young children in the clinic and in the community.

Presented in two main parts, the book explores Nahir Bonifacino's work with children and their parents. The first part presents clinical case material from her work with several young children with an autism spectrum disorder diagnosis, illustrating an adaptation of child psychoanalytic technique that encourages patient communication. Part 2 considers outreach in the community, with resources for parents and professionals in frontline care roles that focus on a preventative approach to child mental health. The book closes with an appendix which translates psychoanalytic resources for use in early childhood education and care institutions.

Psychoanalysis and Severe Disorders in Young Children will be of great interest to child psychoanalysts and psychoanalytic psychotherapists, clinical and educational psychologists, child psychiatrists, social workers, teachers and carers.

Nahir Bonifacino is a child and adolescent psychoanalyst based in Uruguay. She holds a PhD in perinatal and infant psychology and psychopathology and is a member of the Uruguayan Psychoanalytical Association and the International Psychoanalytical Association.

The International Psychoanalytical Association Current Challenges in Psychoanalysis Series
Series Editor: Silvia Flechner
IPA Publications Committee
Natacha Delgado, Nergis Güleç, Thomas Marcacci, Carlos Moguillansky,
Rafael Mondrzak, Angela M. Vuotto, Gabriela Legorreta (consultant)

Recent titles in the Series include:

Psychoanalysis and Severe Disorders in Young Children
Clinical and Community Work with Autism Spectrum Disorder
and Child Mental Health
Nahir Bonifacino

Psychoanalysis and Severe Disorders in Young Children

Clinical and Community Work with Autism Spectrum Disorder and Child Mental Health

Nahir Bonifacino

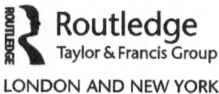
Routledge
Taylor & Francis Group

LONDON AND NEW YORK

Designed cover image: Getty | mgstudyo

First published 2025
by Routledge
4 Park Square, Milton Park, Abingdon, Oxon OX14 4RN

and by Routledge
605 Third Avenue, New York, NY 10158

Routledge is an imprint of the Taylor & Francis Group, an informa business

British Library Cataloguing-in-Publication Data
A catalogue record for this book is available from the British Library

ISBN: 978-1-032-61481-6 (hbk)
ISBN: 978-1-032-61478-6 (pbk)
ISBN: 978-1-032-61482-3 (ebk)

DOI: 10.4324/9781032614823

Typeset in Palatino
by Apex CoVantage, LLC

Contents

Series editor's foreword

Silvia Flechner

The Publications Committee of the International Psychoanalytic Association is delighted to introduce a new addition to our Current Challenges in Psychoanalysis series: *Psychoanalysis and Severe Disorders in Young Children, Clinical and Community Work with Autism Spectrum Disorder and Child Mental Health*. This book, focusing on clinical and community work, is particularly relevant to the work of psychoanalysts, child psychologists, educators and individuals interested in child mental health.

Nahir Bonifacino, PhD, Montevideo, Uruguay, editor and writer of this volume, is an experienced child psychoanalyst in Uruguay and Latin America. She is also well-known in Spain, where she teaches every year. She is involved in teams that care for health and education, caring for infants, young children and their parents and guardians. In her clinical work and research, she observed an increased demand for consultations, including difficulties in verbal communication, emotional expression and social skills. These clinical manifestations are included in several psychopathological conditions such as autism spectrum disorders, Asperger's syndrome and pervasive developmental disorder. Different disciplines, such as neurologists and neuroscience, incorporate distinct visions about this matter. The other important field includes bonding exchanges between parents and infants.

This fascinating book has a first part dedicated to Nahir's clinical practice, "Psychoanalytic clinic: approach to young children with autistic spectrum disorder," and a second part devoted to "Psychoanalysis and community" contributions to an interdisciplinary approach to risk detection and promotion of early emotional development.

As Nahir explains to us,

In recent decades, the rise of Autism Spectrum Disorders in early childhood has become a significant concern for professionals working with young children and their families. This is an important and highly topical issue that affects the mental health of young people and adults of future generations, and that has and will continue to have repercussions for society as a whole.

The depth with which Nahir treats her clinical cases deserves thoughtful reading. Her clinical approach to young children with a diagnosis of autism spectrum disorder shows her commitment to her patients. On the other hand, psychoanalytic outreach to the community offers resources to professionals from related disciplines who are in the first line of care of infants and their parents to foment a preventive approach to child mental health.

I feel honoured to foreword this book due to my relationship with the author. Nahir, a psychoanalyst with whom I have worked, shows her sensitivity and ability to make clear that she is a warm and approachable person at all levels.

Silvia Flechner
Series Editor
Chair IPA Publications Committee

Acknowledgements

I would like to thank psychoanalyst Cristina López de Caiafa, member of the Uruguayan Psychoanalytical Association, for reading the chapters of this book and for sharing her experiences of practising child psychoanalysis.

I would also like to acknowledge the support and contributions I have received from my Uruguayan colleagues Marina Altmann and Ricardo Bernardi, from Robert Emde and Peter Fonagy in the IPA Research Training Programme in 2009, and from Antoine Guedeney in the preventative work and promotion of children's mental health presented in Part 2. Special thanks go to the paediatricians, family doctors and other professionals whose participation and commitment enabled this approach to be implemented in public health centres in Uruguay, and in particular to the paediatrician María Nauar, without whom none of this work would have been possible: as a member of the Technical Advisory Team of the Children's Area of the Primary Care Network of the State Health Services, she took the necessary steps to ensure everything was in place.

Finally, I am grateful to my colleagues, who on different occasions have commented on the clinical material that forms the chapters of the present book, and to the publications committee of the International Psychoanalytic Association, coordinated by Silvia Flechner, for their confidence in this project.

Acknowledgements

Introduction

In recent decades, the rise of autism spectrum disorders in early childhood has become a major concern for professionals from various disciplines who work with young children and their families. This is an important and highly topical issue that affects the mental health of young people and adults of future generations and that has and will continue to have repercussions for society as a whole.

As a child analyst, and perhaps due to a long history of professional involvement with and having formed part of health and education teams that provide care to infants and young children and their parents, in recent years I have experienced increase demand for consultations concerning young children who present with significant difficulties in communication, emotional expression and social skills, among other manifestations of entity.

To a greater or lesser extent and with varying intensity, these clinical manifestations are common to a wide range of severe psychopathological conditions, which the fifth edition of the *Diagnostic and Statistical Manual of Mental Disorders* (*DSM-5*, American Psychiatric Association, 2013) identifies as autism spectrum disorders (ASD). This category includes early childhood autism, Asperger's syndrome and pervasive developmental disorder (PDD), among others. These conditions are now described on the basis of deficits in the functions of communication and social interaction, which has brought them to the attention of the field of neuropaediatrics. For this reason, in recent years it is professionals in this field who establish the differential diagnosis of these children. In general, their treatment approach is based on a protocol that is for the most part aimed at retraining the functions considered to be deficient, that is, verbal communication and motor skills, with or without the intervention of a child psychiatrist.

From another perspective, and with a psychodynamic approach arising from contemporary psychoanalytic theories of development, the *Psychodynamic Diagnostic Manual, 2nd Edition* (PDM-2, Lingiardi and McWilliams, 2017) moves away from a symptomatic behavioural nosography, instead

DOI: 10.4324/9781032614823-1

proposing a multidimensional diagnosis. Based on this conception, emotional development, sensory and regulatory processing capacities, as well as relational patterns and disorders and neurological assessment are crucial components for a multiaxial diagnosis of early childhood disorders (Speranza et al., 2018).

At the same time, current contributions from the neurosciences recognise that early development cannot be conceived in isolation from experience and that sensory, motor and *affective exchanges* of the parent-infant bond during the infant's first year have an impact on structural and functional aspects of development, promoting psychic, emotional, cognitive and social processes that enable the child to live in society (Insel and Young, 2001; Shore, 2001; Fox et al., 2010; Worthman et al., 2010). For several years, early language researchers have also identified gestures, actions and *rhythmic and modulated* vocalisations that develop between mother and baby in a *framework of affective attunement* as protolinguistic forms of communication, which are considered precursors of verbal communication and essential for social development and language (Bloom, 1993; Lam-Cassettari and Kohlhoff, 2020).

These contributions from different disciplines do not conflict with a psychoanalytic perspective that recognises the impact of early bonds on the individual's history. On the contrary, the knowledge emerging from current scientific discoveries concerning early development and the biological correlate of the bonding exchanges between the parents and the infant can enrich and even consolidate our resources for the benefit of the children with whom we are concerned.

This book does not attempt to address the question of the aetiology of severe childhood disorders. Nor is it my intention to provide a historical perspective on the psychoanalytic approach to early autistic disorders.

Instead, this book contains two clearly delimited sections, corresponding to my experience in two areas of psychoanalytic intervention relating to the subject matter at hand. On the one hand, it is a clinical approach to young children who have come to my practice with a diagnosis of autism spectrum disorder. On the other, it constitutes psychoanalytic outreach to the community, offering resources to professionals from related disciplines who are in the first line of care of infants and their parents, to foment a preventive approach to child mental health.

Based on this proposal, the first section of the book is devoted to clinical practice and bears the title "Psychoanalytic clinic. Approach to young children with Autistic Spectrum Disorder". In it, through a range of clinical material about different patients and stages of analytical processes, I illustrate an adaptation of the technique of child psychoanalysis that has favoured communication and encounters with my patients in my clinical practice, as well as their evolution.[1]

Therapeutic approaches in dealing with young children with severe disorders vary widely among analysts, as do ideas of whether or not to incorporate work with parents as part of the child's analytic process. In my experience, an active positioning on the part of the analyst in the search for an encounter with the child, as well as the vicissitudes within the transference-countertransference pair, and the proximity of the parents to the treatment and the evolution of the patient have been essential elements in the approach to the cases which I have treated.

From this perspective, the first chapter of this section dedicated to clinical practice presents the analytical process of a girl who arrived at the clinic at the age of 3, with a diagnosis of pervasive developmental disorder. This work received recognition in the form of the *Rebeca Grinberg Award for Child and Adolescent Psychoanalysis* of the Madrid Psychoanalytic Society, in its first edition in 2017. Then, in Chapter 2, the theoretical-clinical dialogue is gone into in more depth on the basis of references to the analytic process of two other young children who came to my practice between the ages of 2 and 3. This chapter contains an article published in an earlier version in the *International Journal of Psychoanalysis*, 2023.

Chapter 3, in contrast, describes a brief intervention with a 15-month-old baby at risk of autism and her mother, which was carried out based on psychoanalytic contributions to the study of and approach to early bonding difficulties.

Subsequently, Chapter 4 deals with the impact of technology on the early psyche and on the process of subjectivation based on the clinical material of two children aged 2 and a few months old respectively who came to my office with a diagnosis of Autism Spectrum Disorder, presenting a strong attraction to videos and video games.

Finally, ending this clinical section, I present aspects of the technique relating to the analyst's play as a creative resource in the encounter with the child (Chapter 5), the analyst's work with the parents as an important element in the treatment of young children with severe disorders (Chapter 6) and some reflections on the termination of the analytic process of the patients concerned (Chapter 7).

Moreover, in the second section of this book, psychoanalysis is presented beyond its traditional clinical setting and in a community outreach to strengthen the resources of the professionals closest to the babies and their parents for the benefit of early emotional developmental care and infant mental health.

The title of this section is "Psychoanalysis and community. Contributions to an interdisciplinary approach to risk detection and promotion of early emotional development". It describes and analyses various aspects of the work that won a *Psychoanalysis in the Community Award*, subsection Health, of the International Psychoanalytic Association in 2019. This is an initiative that in its initial stages received a grant from IPA and FEPAL to participate as a research project in the *Research Training Programme* at the University of London in 2009, and in 2010 and 2012 received IPA Grants for research.

In this work, psychoanalytic contributions on Early Emotional Development (Winnicott, 1960) are transposed to an operational level in order to generate a dialogue with paediatrics and related professions, promoting a more integrated concept of child health, in which the impact of early bonds in the process of subjectivation and in the development of the newborn's potential capacities is recognised.

The first chapter of this section (Chapter 8) refers to the profound changes that occur in the woman's psyche on experiencing motherhood as determinants of a transferential dynamic between mother, infant and doctor, which turns the paediatric visit into an intervention opportunity for early bonding and infant mental health care.

The following chapter (Chapter 9), titled "Infant withdrawal: a key sign of risk in early emotional development", focuses instead on the infant, and specifically on the analysis of infant withdrawal as a primary defence in the face of sustained difficulties in mother-infant dyad emotional attunement. As has been historically studied by various psychoanalytic authors, it is an early reaction of disengagement or disconnection by the infant, which interferes with early intersubjective experiences and thus with the process of subjectivation.

Chapter 10 of this section then describes the suggested training for health teams in order for them to be able to detect withdrawal early on and promote early emotional development during paediatric appointments, the objective being a preventive approach to infant mental health, starting with the newborn. To conclude the account of this experience, Chapter 11 describes the process of training professionals in a public health centre located in an area of high psychosocial risk in Montevideo (Uruguay), as well as its effects on clinical practice and on infants and their parents.

This work recieved in 2023 the 1st Mention of the X Prize of Infant and Youth Mental Health Research organized by the Child and Adolescent Psychopathology and Mental Health Journal and supported by the city council of Sant Boi de Llobregat, Barcelona, Spain.

Finally, in the form of an appendix (Chapter 12), the resources of psychoanalysis reach the educational field, in order to generate a culture of primary prevention in early bonding and infant mental health in the early childhood education and care institutions, which could constitute a contribution by our discipline to public policymaking.

Note

1 Ethical standards, confidentiality and data anonymity have been respected in the presentation of the clinical material.

References

American Psychiatric Association, DSM-5 Task Force. (2013). *Diagnostic and statistical manual of mental disorders: DSM-5™* (5th ed.). American Psychiatric Publishing, Inc. https://doi.org/10.1176/appi.books.9780890425596

Bloom, L. (1993). *The transition from infancy to language: Acquiring the power of expression*. New York: Cambridge University Press.

Fox, S., Levitt, P. and Nelson, C. (2010). How the timing and quality of early experiences influence the development of brain architecture. *Child Development, 81*(1), 28–40.

Insel, T. and Young, L. (2001). The neurobiology of attachment. *Nature Reviews Neuroscience, 2*(2), 129–136.

Lam-Cassettari, C. and Kohlhoff, J. (2020). Effect of maternal depression on infant-directed speech to prelinguistic infants: Implications for language development. *PLoS One, 15*(7), e0236787. https://doi.org/10.1371/journal.pone.0236787.

Lingiardi, V. and McWilliams, N. (Eds.). (2017). *Psychodinamic diagnostic manual* (2nd ed.; PDM-2). New York: The Gildford Press.

Shore, A. (2001). Effects of a secure attachment relationship on right brain development, affect regulation and infant mental health. *Infant Mental Health Journal, 22*, 7–66.

Speranza, A. M., Malberg, N. and Steele, M. (2018). Mental health and developmental disorders in infancy and early childhood: The PDM-2. *Psychoanalytic Psychology, 35*(3), 328–338.

Winnicott, D. (1960 [1981]). Theory of the parent-infant relationship. In *The maturational process [and the facilitating environment]* (Spanish ed.). Barcelona: Laia.

Worthman, C., Plotsky, P., Schechter, D. and Cummings, C. (2010). *Formative experiences: The interaction of caregiving, culture, and developmental psychobiology*. Cambridge: Cambridge University Press.

Part I

Psychoanalytic clinic

Approach to young children with autistic spectrum disorder

1 From psychic precariousness to subjectivation. The analytical process of a young girl[1,2]

1 *Rebeca Grinberg Prize for Child and Adolescent Psychoanalysis, first edition (2017). The Madrid Psychoanalytical Association.*
2 *Paper published in Spanish in the Revista de la Asociación Psicoanalítica* de Madrid 2017. *No. 81* (Bonifacino, 2017).

This chapter prioritises the clinical account, highlighting the value of child psychoanalysis in achieving psychic structuring and subjectivation in early childhood patients when these processes have been disrupted by significant failures in the primary bonds.

The subject is approached through the analytical process of a little girl, whom I shall call Matilde. She was brought to the clinic at the age of 3. She presented with severe difficulties in psychic functioning, with significant impairment of her motor skills and verbal expression.

I shall place special emphasis on the first stage of the process, in which exchanges deeply imbued with non-verbal elements acquired particular value within the transferential bond and led to an opening of meanings that favoured the development of progressive psychic complexity in the girl. I am referring here to the quality of looks, tone of voice, gestures, mimicry, physical postures and certain playful or non-playful activities in which bodily contact played a part.

I shall go on to give an account of certain milestones in the process and of a final session which took place three and a half years after the first one. This will demonstrate the increasing psychic structuring which enabled Matilde to progress into the typical ups and downs of infantile neurosis.

Initial contacts

Interview with the parents

Matilde's parents are a middle-aged couple who show a certain affective distance. They tell me their daughter is 3 years old and has been attending

DOI: 10.4324/9781032614823-3

school for a year and that the teacher has noticed that she has difficulty communicating.

They say they work long hours and that, before starting school, Matilde was looked after at home by a member of the family's staff.

"Mati didn't want us to leave and cried," they say, "and we would often sneak out unnoticed." The mother tells me that she sometimes had to travel for work, and the father says these occasions were "a chaos of crying and crying without stopping. The child searched all over the house for her mother". They say that when Matilde wakes up they have already left home, and the maid "feeds her and takes her to school by van, and she falls asleep on the way". No details from her first few months of infancy come up. I have the impression that the parents cannot recall them. In response to my question, the mother says that she breastfed for three months during her maternity leave. When various issues come up in the conversation, the husband and wife strongly accuse each other of paying too little attention to the child or of not taking good enough care of her. Both agree that Matilde has not received much attention.

The parents' narrative gave me the impression of a child who seemed to be very lonely and cut off from the possibility of participating in family life. But at the same time, I was struck by her vital drive, which led her to cry, to protest and to demand her mother's presence during her repeated absences.

Interviews with Matilde

Matilde arrives at the first interview with her mother and does not greet me. Neither does she look at me.

She enters the consulting room, and her mother, on her own initiative, stays in the waiting room. I leave the door ajar. I am struck by the distance between the mother and her daughter, who is still young. The girl stands still and says, "All the trees have fallen. All the trees are going to fall like this."

Her expressionless gaze straight ahead, rigid gestures and stereotyped limb movements are striking. I find her appearance and stance touching and at the same time unsettlingly alienating.

Suddenly, I hear her very softly humming a melody that I recognise as coming from a children's rhyme. I stand in front of her, at her level, and begin to sing softly, looking at her and accompanying her tune: "Eensy-weensy spider climbed up the waterspout." There is a moment of encounter between the two of us: Matilde looks at me for the first time and timidly goes on with the melody, while I continue to supply the words: "The rain came down and washed the spider out, the sun came out and dried up all the rain and eensy-weensy spider climbed up the spout again." She then utters some fragmented words and phrases, from which I discern the words "a nest that broke" and "the broken egg of a little bird". On picking up the play material, everything becomes scattered. She talks about the "moon", "stars above", "robot".

Finally, she refers to "a little sheep that wants to be with its mother" and "sheep that want to drink milk next to their mother, next to their father". She also mentions "poo for eating", indicating her confusion, or she uses words that I cannot understand.

"Mati sat down to think," she says. "I did sit down, but I broke down, I broke down. Yes, I did," she adds, staring into space.

The encounter with Matilde causes me great anguish. At times I cannot understand her words or interpret the meaning or intention of her movements. Throughout the first interviews, she continues to create chaos and scatter play equipment around and make references to things being burnt and destroyed. She occasionally utters loose, disjointed sentences with noticeable syntactic flaws and uses words with a meaning of her own. She says, for example, "I'm drinking coffee. It tipped over. I tipped over. But it was Matilde."

In the second interview, after she has once again scattered modelling clay around while trying to use it, I hear her say in a low voice: "Knows the spider." "Who knows the spider?" I ask, crouching down in front of her, so as to meet her gaze. Met with her silence, I myself affirm: "Matilde knows 'the spider', Nahir (analyst's name) knows 'the spider'", and I once more begin to softly sing the children's rhyme that we both know and shared at the beginning. I also tell her that maybe she feels like a little spider that needs to climb up, to become sort of attached to Nahir (the analyst's name), in order to grow. "Yes, attached," Matilde answers, but I doubt how much sense my words will make to her.

"Because Mati's ovenbird broke," she says before we say goodbye, "the ovenbird's nest", and adds, in a low voice, "Mummy". I sense her need for a space like a nest that won't break and in which she can get help to grow, and I tell her so.

First impressions

Matilde introduces herself by talking about things that have fallen and predicting new falls that are bound to happen: "All the trees are going to fall like this." I think that she perceives herself as "falling" and as having a poor holding framework. She feels that her containing framework is too feeble. The scattering of material, the disjointedness of her sentences, her speaking in the third person and the manifestation of uncontainable destructive impulses were evidence of a lack of integration of psychic processes (Winnicott, 1962). The encounter that took place in the first session due to the children's tune allows me an inkling that certain elements were beginning to thread together, such as the melody and words of the song. I consider that the active modality on my part arose in response to my perception that in her precarious psychic state, Matilde could only express isolated and unconnected contents, sketches, like snatches of a melody, and required another to actively offer representations so that these contents could begin to be psychically linked together (Bonifacino, 2014).

"Knows the spider," she says in the second session, after scattering materials about again. Had that encounter been registered as an experience of organisational value? Could this reference be an expression of her expectation of a renewed encounter that, through shared knowledge, could rescue her from distressing and threatening experiences? (Winnicott, 1967). Matilde showed great difficulty in symbolically linking representations and communicating her experiences. However, to the extent that she could perceive me as an emotionally available figure, she was able to convey her suffering, her helplessness and an expectation of encounter – "a little sheep that wants to be with its mother" and "sheep that want to drink milk next to their mother, next to their father" – and of being given something as warm, vital and primary as milk.

The therapeutic indication

The seriousness of the situation and the complexity of its presentation led me to question myself in terms of which aspects to favour in my approach. Although one option was to attend to the functions that appeared to be altered in her development and to proceed with interdisciplinary work, at the same time, the affective distancing shown by her parents in the initial interview and the subsequent meeting with the child led me to favour the communication failures in the early bonds and their impact on Matilde's psychic functioning. From this perspective, the proposal to begin analytical treatment was an attempt to generate, in the affective proximity of the transference framework, certain conditions that were necessary to encourage Matilde's processes of symbolisation and subjectivation, which require a bond to an affectively significant other (Bonifacino, 2014). In this sense, I saw the characteristics of language and the difficulties manifested at a physical level as ego functions which had been affected and interrupted by difficulties in the representational or symbolisation processes, which have their basis in early bonds.

The initial proposal was to offer biweekly sessions, regular interviews with parents, and contact with the school and the teacher. This framework gave me time to evaluate the possibilities of analytical work with Matilde and the commitment that the parents were able to take on and to think about proceeding with interdisciplinary work. The parents accepted my proposal. The positive evolution of the girl a few months after starting treatment led to a frequency of three weekly sessions, which was maintained for three years until the end of treatment.

Psychic precariousness

> An infant who has no one person to gather his bits together starts with a handicap in his own self-integrating task, and perhaps he cannot succeed, or at any rate cannot maintain integration with confidence.
>
> Winnicott, 1945. *Primitive emotional development*

First session: An encounter

In the first session, Matilde runs in without looking at me. Her arms move stiffly at the sides of her body. She goes to the table where the materials are kept. Sitting on a chair, she separates out small pieces of modelling clay while uttering some expressions without any context: "from the fireplace", "with that plate". I sit next to her and describe her actions, assuming they contain a certain intentionality:

A: "You're playing with modelling clay. Let me see? What do you want to do with it?" Matilde does not look at me but makes a little ball of modelling clay. I offer her the palm of my hand, and she places the ball in it.

M: "It's a little ball. I'm going to make a big ball." She then places this on my hand too, while many little pieces of modelling clay fall and scatter.

A: "The little ball and the big ball are together and held," I say, looking at her and looking for a moment at the little balls of modelling clay in my hand. "Just as you and I are together in this place, getting to know each other and working together, so that you can feel better."

M: "A snake, another snake, for the little snakes," she says, while trying to make a "little snake" out of modelling clay. She then models something else and adds, "The mother and her little child."

A: "The mother and her little child are together."

M: "Yes, why not. Food she's going to the food." While saying this, she gazes at the floor and makes stereotypical movements with her hands.

A: "Is she going to eat?"

M: "She's hungry."

A: "Maybe, like the little child, the little daughter Mati is hungry, hungry for words. Hungry to understand the things that you feel."
Matilde lifts her face, looks me in the eye for the first time in the session, and asks me, "What's your name?"

A: "My name is Nahir, and your mum and dad told me that your name is Matilde. It is important to get to know each other, and it is also important for you to get to know yourself. And together we are going to get to know what you feel, what you want, what you think, the things that happen to you."

Putting things into words, giving meaning, helping her to organise her disorganised or chaotic scene was to be my constant function during the early stages of the process. Offering her ways to link or even to build things that she could only express in fragmented form was a way to work towards organising her inner world. Here we are, the two of us, in our first session and initiating an encounter, in which her "hunger" and needs are recognised.

Second session: exploring

> I wanted to describe the world, because to live in a non-described world was too lonely.
>
> N. KRAUSS, 2005. *The History of Love.*

Matilde runs in, without looking at me. She goes to her box and unexpectedly knocks the lid off and steps on it with a great lack of control. I rest my hand on the lid, preventing her from breaking it, and look her in the eye.

A: "No, Mati. We're going to take care, we're going to take care of your box, we're going to take care of the things for our work here, and I'm also going to take care of you and me." She frowns at me.

A: "Ooh! You are showing me that you are angry!" I point out, in a projected and particularly serious tone of voice, exaggerating my own frown.

   Matilde takes a marker and throws it hard, explosively pulling and scattering bits of modelling clay.

A: "When you get angry, you feel a very big scattering in you. You are showing me this big scattering so that I can help you."

   She stops and looks at me. She then looks at the brown marker on the table and, pointing to it, says,

M: "It's the brown one."

A: "When the strong anger passes, when you no longer feel that you are in bits, then you can say what it is: it's the brown one," I say to her, looking at her.

   Matilde makes a line with the marker on a sheet of paper, and when I ask her what it is, she answers,

M: "A little snail."

A: "Maybe that little snail needs a big snail to take care of it, so that it doesn't feel it is in pieces, so it can be protected from the strong feelings it might have."

   She draws some more lines.

A: "What is it?"

M: "Ghost! Woo! Woo! A monster!" she answers restlessly, her voice raised, making messy strokes. Meanwhile, she abruptly and disconnectedly mentions, "A TV cartoon, a doll, pee-pee and poo." Then she throws more bits of modelling clay and suddenly throws the ball hard at me.

A: "Woo!" I say, exaggerating her intonation. "You are showing me all the powerful and tangled things that you feel, and which suddenly scare you a lot, like monsters and ghosts!"

Matilde looks at me, moves to the couch, and sits down next to a section of the couch where the sun is shining in through the window. She gently moves her hand towards the brighter patch and touches it slowly and repeatedly. I go up to her and say, "You're touching the warmth. It's a nice feeling, it's pleasant." She looks at me and then continues to touch nearby surfaces, as if exploring sensations of warmth and less warmth. She seems calm. I try to go along with her explorations. I touch the surfaces after her each time, placing my hand close to hers. I also look at her and convey my perception: "This one's warm too, isn't it?" In response, Matilde looks at me and nods shyly. In contrast, when the surface is warmer, she withdraws her hand quickly and looks at me expectantly, waiting for gestures and words. "Phew! And this one is almost burning," I say at such times, also quickly withdrawing my hand. She then looks at different objects. Each time she looks at me, she looks at the object, points to it with her index finger so I look at it, and asks, "And this?" She waits for words that identify what she points to each time. In this way Matilde points at the armchair, the lamp, the clock, etc., one after the other, and I name them.

At the end of this activity, she goes to the room where her mother is and takes her by the hand. Her mother is sitting in an armchair, while I express the invitation that the child has extended to her. Matilde crawls under the armchair where her mother is sitting and rolls herself in the foetal position. I look at her and say, "It's as if you were inside Mummy!" Leaving this space, she climbs up her mother's body until she is sitting on her lap. From there, she insistently slides her hands over her mother's body and face. Although her mother initially tolerates this close contact, she becomes uncomfortable and gently removes her hands. "Matilde needs to feel very close to Mummy, but Mummy also helps her to grow when she invites her to look for other ways of being together," I say.

The establishment of precise and consistent limits on my part was having a protective effect on the child against the perception of uncontrollable impulses that caused her an intense feeling of fragmentation. At times, the boundaries generated fierce anger, but they gradually took on a holding effect and an organising value. The proposal to take care – of her box, the space, to take care of ourselves – is not intended to deny the destructive impulses that inhabit the patient, but rather to welcome them within a framework of containment, which enables her to function differently. From the recognition and containment of these impulses, and the identification of her experiences of lack of protection against them, Matilde can set out within the analytical framework to explore her immediate environment and to discover sensations and objects, with the expectation of naming and signifying.

Elements as primary as the sensations themselves were presented to be named and discerned, enabling a progression towards appropriation of them as subjective experiences. Her affects were also being identified and verbalised: "You got angry." At the same time, exchanges deeply imbued with non-verbal elements occupied a central and sustained place at the start of the process. The look, the mimicry, the gestures and the different tones of voice that arose spontaneously on my part and accompanied the affects in play were opening her senses, encouraging expressions of increasing complexity in the child. In the last part of the session, the exploratory movement extends to the mother figure. I understand the transition from the foetal position to this close contact with her mother's body to be Matilde's expectation of a new encounter, which within the analytic framework could give rise to a new birth: her birth as a psychic subject.

Session 3: unifying

> In between the infant and the object is some thing, or some activity or sensation. In so far as this joins the infant so the object . . . so far is this the basis of symbol-formation.
>
> (Winnicott, 1960, p. 176)

Matilde brings five lollipops. She asks me to unwrap them and puts them all in her mouth at once. I tell her no, that they go in her mouth one at a time, because otherwise she might hurt herself, and I remind her that we are going to take care that she doesn't hurt herself. She looks at me, takes them out of her mouth, and says the colour of one of them. I tell her to show me that she knows the colours, and together we identify the colour of each of the others. I then ask her which colour she likes best, and she picks up the red lollipop and shows it to me. I name the colour of the lollipop and also tell her which one I like best. I expressly choose another one – the blue one – which I also pick up and show to her. Then, I say, projecting my voice as if it were my own blue lollipop, which I position in front of her red lollipop:

A: "Hello, red lollipop, how are you?"
    Matilde looks at me, smiles, and moves her lollipop, as I had just done with mine.
A: "They are greeting each other," I tell her, in my own tone of voice, and looking at her with a certain complicity.
    To my surprise, she looks at me and adds:
M: "They are lollipop puppets."
    I find her response very stimulating. I understand that we are slipping into a symbolic universe. Is this the start of a certain possibility of play? Matilde then puts her lollipop in her mouth.

A: "Ah! The lollipop is gone! Where is the red lollipop, I can't see it?" I ask, searching and looking around. "Lollipop? Where are you?" Matilde looks at me and smiles. She is happy, but not excited. Suddenly, she pulls the lollipop out of her mouth and shows it to me, looking at me expectantly. I gesture in surprise.

A. "It's reappeared!! There you are, lollipop!" I say, looking at it, and then, looking at Matilde, I add: "Naughty lollipop! It was hiding!" Matilde enjoys this activity very much and repeatedly puts the lollipop in her mouth and resumes this hide-and-seek sequence over and over again. Perhaps with some over-enthusiasm or testing the consistency of the boundaries, she again tends to put all the lollipops in her mouth at the same time. I avert this. I tell her no, and I tell her again that she could get hurt that way. I also tell her that I think she is very pleased with this game, and that she is probably very eager to continue playing, but that we cannot play with all the lollipops in her mouth at once.

She looks at me and listens to me. She then makes the lollipops roll down the slope of the couch, so that they roll and slip as if on a slide. My tone of voice is somewhat enthusiastic as I verbalise along with each go on the slide: "The lollipop is having a go on the slide!" Standing at the other end of the couch, I catch each one, preventing them from falling to the floor. After repeated goes, she herself climbs onto the couch and tries to slide down, turning and repeating the route that the lollipops had taken so far. I help her in this initiative, verbalise her journey, sitting at the other end of the couch. Each time I wait for her, as I had done for the lollipops, holding her to prevent her from falling. She enjoys the physical contact and laughs in amusement. I notice that a certain vitality is beginning to awaken in Matilde. She enjoys the sensations, the anticipation of her journey and the certainty of being held. I accompany the development with words – sometimes descriptive, sometimes interpretative: "Ooh! How frightening! She's falling, falling. Mati?! Oh no!!!" I say, as I hold her in my arms. "You're having so much fun! We are playing and having a lot of fun together."

In this session, Matilde builds an elaborate lollipop object. An object that also refers to the oral, to basic, primary and vital sensations. She precariously constructs her own bodily schema from the different sensations that are unified in the object. This gives rise to an elementary experience of herself as a unit. Primary bodily sensations and experiences are explored in the analytical space: touch, taste, kinaesthesia in the turning and sliding on the couch, holding, and the gaze that confirms the constancy of the object in the game of "it's there, it's gone." For a long time, Matilde insisted in repeatedly turning around on the couch and being caught by me just before she fell. This led to a series of enjoyable exchanges between us. Even during later, more advanced stages of the process, she resorted to this game when she was feeling especially anxious, or when confronted with experiences that threatened her psychic integration. Furthermore, this way of repeating shared experiences, which gradually became threaded through with subtle variations, also provided a secure and containing framework. Only on a basis of monotony can [a mother] profitably add richness (Winnicott, 1945).

Symbolising. Subjectifying

At first, some of Matilde's actions had taken place on a concrete level. For example, she tended to actually eat the dough when talking about "baby food", or when making a snake out of modelling clay, she was very scared, fearful it would attack her. Recognising, giving meaning and designating what she was doing enabled symbolic processes to emerge. At the end of the first month, she begins to verbalise affection through fragments of the words of a song that is very popular among girls her age. "Co . . . co . . . co . . . I love you . . ." she sings happily, while tracing on the blackboard. She looks at me and says, "A flower, and it seems to be for you." Affection and gratitude were beginning to flow in elementary forms, and words were emerging as a means of conveying experiences. Certain ideas of care were also emerging. In the second month of analysis, she asks me to cut something out, and watching my actions steadily, she would say: "Watch your fingers, watch your fingers, Nahir!" The actions of caring and repairing directed at the object – and at the self at the same time (Klein, 1940a) – were signs of the emergence of certain ego-functions. Gradually, more representative activities appeared. She asks me to draw for her "a little house, a car and a baby". Later, she says, "It's Matilde." Her world was beginning to be enriched with words, and to be populated by objects and people from school and her family, which she identified by name. She was also beginning to show her intentionality by anticipating what she was going to do: "I'm going to play with this lid, I'm going to make a snail," she said, later adding excitedly: "I did it!" At the same time, notions of time (the time implicit in the anticipation of her action) and space (graphic space), the object and the self, were being constructed (Klein, 1940b).

As her representational skills increased, difficulties in structuring language gradually began to subside, and her movements became less rigid. Matilde was taking possession of her body. However, important oscillations in its functioning persisted. Sessions with symbolic displays and a tendency towards integration coexisted with others in which the destructive, disjointed, and muddled contents emerged unchecked at a frenetic pace, aspects which were for the most part partial and fragmented. Disorganisation set in, and words lost their communicative potential. Such sessions occurred more frequently at the beginning of the process. I found them overwhelming and felt they raised enormous doubt about the child's prognosis.

I shall attempt to convey a snippet from one of these sessions, although any attempt to transcribe the events of a segment of the session implies a mediation of sequences and words that dampens the impact of the chaotic and dizzying nature of its content by superimposing a certain order and illation.

In the air

In a session three months into the analysis, Matilde comes running in, with a downward gaze, her arms held stiffly and tensely at her sides. Her movements are jerky and particularly uncontrolled. She goes to the table where her box is. I position myself nearby on a small chair.

M: "It's nothing. A sausage." She disdainfully lifts the lid of her box, which falls back. "I'm going to make a heart," she immediately adds. While scribbling on a piece of paper, she says quickly, without pause and in a monotone: "This is not a heart and it's not a bone, nor is it a bone for a dog to eat."

   She has still not looked at me up to this point. I try to draw her attention with questions and in a slow, gentle voice, showing my interest in trying to understand. The distinction between fantasy and reality is precarious in the child at the moment.

A: "Is it a bone, Mati?"

M: "It's a dog biscuit."

   She speaks quickly and without looking at me. She is very restless. Her tense facial expressions have become grotesque and uncontrolled grimaces. This has a strong impact on me. It distresses me and I feel very concerned. I try to summon her back to her expressed intention: drawing the heart.

A: "Is it a dog biscuit? And what happened to the heart?"

M: "Yes, I'm going to make a heart." She moves quickly over to the couch, taking the scissors and coloured paper. "I'm going to make a crayon out of this little brown paper," she says, making quick cuts on several pieces of paper.

   Unexpectedly and explosively, she puts her feet on the wall, making it visibly dirty. She looks at me expressionlessly.

   I try to recover from my surprise and anger. I say, "No, we are going to take care." She insists and tries to repeat this action again and again, now with a defiant look.

   I also insist with words, while repeatedly holding her feet away from the wall and looking at her firmly. Then Matilde seems to stop what she is doing. I breathe a sigh of relief and feel tired. She immediately takes a red paper, kisses it and gives it to me.

A: "That's an affectionate gesture. Maybe it's like saying 'thank you, Nahir, for holding me back and taking care of me'."

M: "I have little pieces of paper. I'm going to make a black heart." With difficulty, she untidily cuts the paper into little pieces while shouting repeatedly and louder and louder: "Ah! Ah! Ah!" At the same time her jerky, stereotypical bodily movements resume.

   I position myself in front of her at her height, and resting my hand on her shoulder to get her to look at me, I say to her, "Well, Mati, today you are showing me that something is going on that makes you very,

very restless. Let's try to understand it, but behaving like that doesn't do you any good." Matilde looks at me and seems to hear me, but she is still very agitated. She rushes around the consulting room in a disorganised to-and-fro. I stand in front of her, stopping her in her tracks. I bend down, hold her arms and tell her not to do that and that I am going to take care of her and of these strong things that are happening to her and that don't make her feel good. She struggles free, runs off again and bumps into an armchair. Even so, she continues on as if in a frenzied whirl, spinning rapidly on her axis and continually intoning a kind of refrain: "[She] flies and flies without stopping! Flies and flies without stopping!!" I feel exhausted. I find it distressing. She seems to be in an uncontrolled state, hurting herself. I hold her again, position myself in front of her at her height, and once more try to calm her with a gentle voice, speaking slowly: "You are showing me that sometimes you feel you are in the air, and there is a very, very big force inside you that won't let you stop and that doesn't make you feel good. And that great force sometimes makes you crash, like when you bumped into the armchair, and you can hurt yourself a lot. It seems to me that you are wanting me to help you to slow down. I'm not going to let you run like this, and I'm not going to let you spin like this either, because it's not good for you."

The girl looks at me and listens. I stop holding her arms. She walks towards the blackboard, and says she is going to draw. In fact, she still lacks control and only succeeds in drawing untidy lines, without managing to make a shape. I tell her that today she is showing me she is spilling out. That today she feels as if she doesn't have a shape or any boundaries and there is nothing keeping her together.

M: "Cutting, curting, knife; cutting, curting, knife," Matilde says repeatedly, picking up a toy knife.

Sometimes Matilde felt she was "nothing" or that she was a flood of uncontrolled impulses which operated independently and of their own accord, with dire consequences for her psychic functioning. In the early days, I felt unconditionally called upon to take on a maternal function of support and psychic organisation. Matilde demanded a great physical and mental effort from me in each session and caused me very ambivalent and intense feelings. This may have been necessary for affects to begin to flow, and for her to be able to get in touch with them. At times, the way she scattered material around and her persistent unruliness made me feel very angry. At other times, I felt discouraged and found myself doubting my analytical resources to work with her. But at the same time, I was moved by her gratitude, I sensed her helplessness, and it caused me great distress when I could no longer understand her functioning, when contact was interrupted and her gaze was lost in empty space, or when I became a mere spectator of certain sequences of psychic disintegration. In the latter situations, it took a great effort on my part to find the resources to bring her back into the analytic bond.

Interview with the parents

Matilde's parents' affectively distant manner manifested as a characteristic feature which extended to other bonds and was difficult to work with. Even so, they were able to sustain the continuity of the process and were receptive to my ideas. A few months after starting, they told me they could see significant changes in the child, which were confirmed by her school. They noted a greater tendency to communicate and that she sought social contact. I felt that perhaps they, too, were beginning to pay their daughter closer attention. In monthly or bimonthly interviews that I requested in the early days, I showed some of Matilde's needs that they were unable to perceive and, as such, also unable to respond to. Also, because of their characteristic functioning, I took the initiative to point out in very concrete terms everyday situations which would make the child feel lonely and abandoned or the lack of organising routines at home, which subjected her to frankly distressing situations. I also conveyed to them Matilde's expectation to share in fun activities with them, such as games and walks.

The favourable evolution of the process shortly after it began – with progressive remission of the symptoms that compromised the child's oral expression and bodily skills – was endorsing the therapeutic strategy proposed and led me to consider a third weekly session. This frequency began eighth months into the work and continued for two years, creating a favourable framework for continuity.

"Making the girl"

Being–not being

> I'm going under the armchair, so you can't see me, but you have to look for me, please.
>
> MATILDE, 4 years old

Six months into our sessions and after the first holiday period, some of Matilde's initiatives led to a game of hide-and-seek. There were several variants which arose at different points in the process and which reflected the configuration of new and more complex psychic frameworks. Matilde stands in front of me, making sure I can see her face, closes her eyes and says, "I have my eyes closed. And now I don't!" she adds, opening them, and quickly getting under the armchair.

A: "Hmmm. Now I'm the one who can't see you," I say in an intrigued tone of voice. And with searching gestures and a playful tone, I add, "Matiii, where are you?"

M: "Under the armchair!" she cheerfully replies.

A: "Ah! We're playing hide-and-seek!"

M: "I'll count, you hide," she proposes, coming out from her hiding place.
    I hide behind an armchair, but I notice that she also goes behind the
    other one, making us mutually invisible.
    I then decide to come out of hiding and look for her, talking expect-
    antly, "Let's see, where is Mati? I can't see her! Where is Matilde
    hiding?"
M: "Here I am!" she says enthusiastically, jumping out in full view with-
    out giving me time to find her.

Matilde was to repeat various forms of this game, which she evidently
found enjoyable, in this and other sessions. Sometimes she would look
for me, imitating my phrases and expectant tone: "Where is Nahir? Where
have you hidden?" until I give some sign from my hiding place that catches
her attention and helps her to find me, to her great satisfaction. At other
times, she says, "Hiding", although she only covers her face, leaving her
body visible. She enjoys this activity. I conveyed what I was perceiving:
"You like to play hide-and-seek. You really like to hide and know that I'm
going to look for you and find you. You like it when we meet up, like when
you arrive and we see each other every day."

Matilde kept asking to be looked for and looked at, which at the same
time was a strong demand for narcissistic libidinisation. In the context of a
strong transferential bond as a backdrop to the process, the realisation that
I had an inexhaustible willingness to look for her, name her and find her was
taking on a structuring value for the child. This play of presence-absence
that expressed her expectation of a closer and more desiring maternal function was to be enriched with new developments in later sessions.

Discovering the body

> For the child, the problem of becoming aware of or open to [the outside
> world] is a false problem . . . the only problem will be rather to close oneself,
> to close a self, or an I, whatever the periphery may be.
>
> (Laplanche, 1989, p. 93)

In a later session, the child arrives and lies face-down on the couch, as if
inert. She does not answer my greeting, nor make any sign at all. I perceive
this as a manifestation of her sense of non-existence. I start to call out to her
and look for her, like the game of hide-and-seek that we started in previous
sessions, and which since then has arisen in every meeting.

A. "Mati, where are you? Where is Matilde, I can't hear her? Let's see if
    I can find her." I approach the couch, and showing surprise, I pat it, as
    if finding different parts of her body: "Ah! But here are Mati's feet. And

here are her legs!" I thus list her back, arms, head, until finally reaching her eyes, at which point I say, generating a certain anticipation: "And where are Matilde's eyes? Let's see if I can see them." She turns her head, looks at me and smiles. She then turns back to face the wall again as she had at the beginning, as is offering to play the same game again, which I accept.

She then goes to the table and draws on the blackboard. She pauses, looks at me and asks me:

M:　"Why don't you draw me a face?"

A:　"It seemed to me that you were going to draw."

M:　"You do it." She gives me the marker, and I start to draw, telling her what I'm doing and asking her about the details:

A:　"Let's see, let's draw a face: the eyes, the nose, the mouth. Shall I draw some hair?" She nods, and I draw it. Then I look at the image, I look at her, and I ask: "Could it be Matilde's face?" She looks at me and nods enthusiastically. Then she looks at her body and asks me to draw the clothes she is wearing: her flowered T-shirt, her striped trousers, her shoes. I perceive that the previous journey through her body while she was on the couch is now perhaps somehow transferred to the drawing on the blackboard. The capacity for representation has been extended to new registers.

M:　"I'm playing in the park," she adds, pointing to a space on the black-board and giving me to understand that I should continue with the drawing, "with clouds and sky and trees and little flowers."

I draw what she asks me to in the position she points to. She is very pleased when she sees the images appear on the blackboard, and at times she shows a certain tension in her limbs. The result is a drawing with a lot of detail and colour. She gets up from her chair and looks at the picture in perspective. She decides to add more details:

M:　"This short hair," she says, pointing to her bangs. I draw it, and she is satisfied: "I'm playing in the park, and there are swings over there," she adds. We both look at the drawing with genuine satisfaction.

A:　"How beautiful you look, Mati, and you're playing!"

M:　"Thank you for you," she says, looking at me and with a very affection-ate gesture, which I find touching. "Thank you for you."

Within the framework of the analytical relationship, Matilde was discover-ing new potentialities. A request to "make the girl", which she said insist-ently at this stage of the work, configured a particular milestone in the processes of psychic integration, and manifested an expectation that went beyond the concrete aspect of the drawing she expected from me: "Will you make me a girl?" she demanded, "come on, a happy girl, will you make me? Please, make me a girl, make me a well-made girl." The configuration of a body schema and the acquisition of language that was beginning to be conjugated in the first person were revealing a process of subjectivation. In the manner of a mirror image, in successive sessions Matilde asked me to draw a picture of the girl, with an outfit that corresponded to the clothes she was wearing on each occasion. "This is me," she would sometimes say. And at the same time, realising the precariousness of her psychic functioning at the end of the session, when I erased the drawing, she would say in an anguished tone: "Why did you erase me?" At each separation, she experienced a discontinuity that erased her own existence and often showed anger and hostility when it was time to say goodbye. "I don't want to go!!" she insisted. Gradually, trust in the bond would give way to an experience of continuity, which cushioned the farewells.

One year into the process, Matilde actively and insistently asked me to look at her drawings, which also implied a need to be looked at herself: "Look!" She was also beginning to express structuring conflicts that are typical of infantile neurosis. Progressively, she developed a naturally avid curiosity about the origin of babies and sexual differences, and the castration fantasy became a source of anguish and anxiety (Freud, 1905, 1908). New appeals to the father figure arose in this discourse. Her discoveries generated surprise and anxiety, and she brought her vitality and mischievousness into play. On one occasion, she said, "The dad and the boy have willies. The girl and the mother have willies. Oh no! I made a mistake! I thought girls and mummies had willies!"

"I have a crown."

> I'm like a baby, because when I haven't got any shoes on I make myself tiny and get in Nahir's one.
> It's like magic – I'm growing!
>
> MATILDE, aged 4

At the age of almost five, Matilde arrives at the session very happy. She looks at me expectantly, opens her mouth and shows me, in her hand, her first tooth which had fallen out. "Ah! You're big," I say enthusiastically. She nods, proudly. She then gives me a drawing she has brought from home. It is a colourful flower that she has drawn herself.

M: "It's in a pot, and these little dots are the soil."
A: "How beautiful! You feel like this beautiful flower when you see yourself growing!" She looks at me and nods. She draws lots of little hearts on a sheet of paper.
A: "What a lot of little hearts!" She draws a huge heart that envelops them: "What a lot of affection! So much love! It seems to me that you want to show me your gratitude, your affection. You feel that the work we are doing here together helps you to grow."

M: "Shall we play kitty? I was the kitten; you were the mother . . . human. You were the human mother." She makes a "crib" by joining two arm-chairs together, as she has done on other occasions. She curls up and covers herself up. She talks to me from there: "I like animals, except tigers and lions. And do you know what colour I don't like? I don't like black, but I like pink, because that's a girl's colour."

She then proposes that we become two princess friends. Like a young princess, she will proudly display certain physical skills, which she happily tells me she learned from her big friend: lifting a chair with one hand, hopping on one foot, etc. She has taken ownership of her physical movements and enjoys them. Before leaving, she gives me the drawing of the flower. On her way out, she places a small box on her head that contains her tooth which has fallen out and leaves singing: "I have a crown! I have a crown!"

Matilde saw herself growing and evolving. She was expressive and vital, and her gestures had become increasingly harmonious and fluent. There were significant developments during sessions. She enjoyed giving me "surprises", in which I only participated by being present at a distance. "Don't look, don't look," she insisted at the time, making drawings that she would later show me with satisfaction. She no longer needed my gaze to be able to create. In the words of Winnicott (1958): "The holding environment is the basis for what gradually becomes a self-experiencing being. . . . In this phase the ego changes over from an unintegrated state to a structured integration" (p. 43).

New meetings with the parents

Encouraged by Matilde's evolution, her parents showed a genuine appreciation of the process. Despite their own difficulties, they were becoming more available to their daughter, whom they were beginning to see as a capable and creative child.

Her mother spontaneously told me about playful activities they were beginning to discover together, such as "playing at sharing a cup of tea".

She also began to share walks with Matilde, who, with evident satisfaction, would refer to them in the session as " women's outings". The child treasured these encounters with her mother and felt that she was taking up her own valued place in the family, which enabled her in her narcissistic libidinisation and sexual identification.

Matilde's father had also brought about some favourable changes and was able to notice the girl's search for him. "She prefers her father," he said proudly, but at the same time, he acknowledged his difficulty in dealing with various situations that subjected his daughter to disorganising experiences. During a certain stage of the process, Matilde demanded a consistent paternal function in the transferential framework.

On ending

Historicising. The caterpillar and the butterfly

In the second year of the process, while drawing Matilde tells me,

M: "It's a butterfly and the little cocoon. But it's already become a butterfly, and here it was when it was a caterpillar."
A: "Maybe you feel that you have changed, like the caterpillar that has become a butterfly."
M: "This is a strange creature. It's a caterpillar, but it looks like a strange creature. We can put on a play, like we did last year. Do you remember? I remember."
A: "Here the strange little caterpillar Mati grew and changed, until she became a butterfly."
M: "What letter does the caterpillar start with?"
A: "C, the round one." I accompany my words with a circular gesture.
M: "Ah! Like a circle." She writes it. "And I'm making a little ring-halo for the butterfly here, because it is an angel butterfly. It's called the angel-butterfly."
A: "Will it be a good little angel butterfly? You have been discovering lots of good things inside you, which have allowed you to grow, to learn, to have friends, to be with mum and dad in a different way." Matilde listens to me, while she calmly and very colourfully draws the caterpillar.
M: "You see? This is the story of the caterpillar and the butterfly. Once upon a time there was a caterpillar. Hold on, I'm making a little book." She picks up two sheets of paper and sticks them together.
A: "Like the little book of this story that we are making together here."
     She tries to write "Once upon a time", asking me for some of the letters. It strikes me that she can clearly identify them when I merely mention them, and I tell her this with evident surprise.
A: "Oh, Mati! How can you recognise so many letters?!"
M: "What?" she says in surprise, in a loud voice, looking at me and stopping her activity for a moment. And as if it were obvious, she goes on: "You taught them to me!"
     She then asks me to write the story she is creating in the book, pausing every now and then to illustrate it.
M: "Once upon a time there was a butterfly that lived in a forest, and a snail." She draws and colours in. "I'll make its mouth. And the grass and the sun here. It was happy. And after they met, they saw a honeycomb, and the bees followed them, and they ran away. There is the butterfly and the snail, and here the little bees." She points at her drawing. "And they fly away, and as the snail was a bit slow, the butterfly carried it."

Matilde shows her command of language, her ability to historicise her analytical process and to think of herself with her own history of change and evolution. Her short-illustrated story tells of being immersed in a symbolic world of letters that make up words, and of words that have taken on meaning through the transference relationship. Could "the slow snail" be a figuration of an aspect of her own that alludes to the perception of her difficulties? A new era was dawning in the process. Through tales and illustrated or acted-out stories, she was showing a degree of psychic structuring and dynamism that allowed for the creative development of fantasies and gave rise to new analytical possibilities. Id impulses were enriching the self (Winnicott, 1958).

The world of colours

> Should we not look for the first traces of imaginative activity as early as in childhood?
>
> FREUD, 1907

In a later session, Matilde goes straight to her box and takes out a cardboard oar that we had made on another occasion. She is very active, standing the two small chairs close together facing each other, saying that it is a boat. She invites me to sit on one of them, and she sits on the other. She then pretends to row and that we are travelling together in the boat. I go along with this game, pointing out what she is doing or sometimes asking questions to better understand her intention or to encourage her to develop her fantasy.

Suddenly, pointing into the distance, she says that there is a shark coming and asks me to start the engine of our boat to go faster. Then, continuing this adventure that she is creating, she says that there are waves coming, and we both row in time as the waves roll the ship. At a certain point, Matilde says we have arrived and that we have to disembark to buy pets. In our scene, she buys a puppy, and at her suggestion, I buy a seahorse. We take them back to the boat and set off. We played and acted out the different episodes of her story together. She then proposed we build an aeroplane, using the material in the consulting room very creatively for this purpose. She gives the impression of working calmly. At her initiative, we now position the chairs that formed the boat one behind the other. She chooses some materials, and we assemble the various parts of the plane: she makes the wings with some cushions, the tail of the plane with the lid of her box, and so on. She also chooses the tables and plates for the food that is going to be served on the trip. She enjoys this activity. At her suggestion, we sit in the plane and travel to another country. We travel downwards together, and she says we are going to go up a hill. She positions large cushions as scenery to give the impression of altitude and adopts a strained expression, as if labouring uphill. She fetches her scissors, which she says can be an axe, and picks up a pencil, which she says can be a "stick". She gestures, pretending to "hitch" these instruments to "the top of the hill". Finally, she makes an accurate throw, which pleases us both as this will allow us to "go uphill". Matilde places the packet of markers on "the summit" and says,

M: "The treasure is up the hill. It's hidden. They were the colours, because there weren't any colours."
      We climbed the hill, making a show of it being hard work. She leads, and I follow. Finally, as if having reached a cherished goal, she says she finds
M: "The colours, which give colour to the world."
      She then takes the packet with the markers and drops them one by one on different places around the consulting room, speaking as she does so:
M: "This one for the land," she says of the brown one: "Blue for the sky. Violet, red and lilac for the little flowers that look pretty. And with this one, the leaves on the trees will turn green." She then invites me to sit next to her and look at the view together: "Now, that the world is in colour," she says.

United and apart

By the end of the third year of the process, there began to be signs that it was nearing termination. Matilde felt more confident in her achievements and abilities and began to show a certain reluctance to attend the sessions. She was centred on her own interests, which were appropriate for her age, and took pleasure in discovering letters and in learning them. In exchanges with her teacher and the school psychologist, they conveyed a picture of a lucid child, liked by her friends and without any difficulties with her schoolwork.

Matilde was 6 years old and well into her first year of primary school when we reached the end of the process. At the last moment she proposed a review of the various activities that we had shared from the beginning. In the penultimate session, she chooses a memory game, which we had not played for a long time.

M: "We also played the lottery with this game we; do you remember?"
A: "Ah! You can remember so much about the things we used to do a long time ago!"
      She recalls comments we used to make about the characters in this game, and then I also add other aspects, which I myself remember.
A: "We can both remember so much! We do have a good memory!" She nods, and I notice that this confirmation is a relief to her. Then, making a scrap of paper appear and disappear under some small cups, she says that she is doing some "magic".
A: "Maybe you'd like to be able to do magic to make me appear like the scrap of paper whenever you feel like it, if ever you miss coming here."

Matilde stands up, almost curtsying with her whole body, opening her arms and bowing her head in a graceful gesture.

M: "Da-dah!" she says musically, projecting her voice, adding: "Hello! I am Nahir!"

She laughs and makes me smile. Then she goes to the blackboard and draws a heart, which she immediately makes "disappear" by erasing it, while saying that it has magical powers.

There are moments when I am pleasantly surprised to see her so unselfconscious, playing creatively, displaying her affects and her fears, and I realise that I also perceive her to be full of "magic".

A: "You are showing me your magical powers of growing, playing, learning and drawing. All this magic which you have now that our work together is ending."

She goes to the blackboard, draws two cherries joined by the stalk and then rubs out the line joining them, leaving them separated.

A: "The cherries Mati and Nahir. United, and now they are going to separate."

She draws her face on one of the cherries, and then mine, highlighting the differences. She makes the mouths round.

M: "They are saying 'owww!'" she explains, "because they had the stick that joins them cut."

A: "Separation also hurts."

M: "Like that, here's the knife, look," she says, drawing a dagger. Then she erases the round mouth on the cherry that represents me and gives it a smile instead. "She's smiling."

A: "Of course, separating hurts, but I am also smiling and I'm happy, because I see that you feel good, and that you have been able to grow, in many, many, ways."

At the top of the board, above the two cherry heads, she writes "separated".

A: "Separated, because you aren't going to come anymore." Underneath she writes "together" and adds a kind of double-headed arrow, which both joins and separates the two cherries. "But together because we are connected by many memories, we share many memories after all this time together."

I suggest putting the things away. Matilde accepts, and as she says goodbye from the doorway, she looks at me, runs back and gives me a heartfelt hug and a kiss.

Personally, I feel very gratified when a patient, especially a young child, can regain his or her "potential capacities" (Winnicott) and take up his or her life creatively. I see the end of the analysis as a joint achievement. In Matilde's case, I was astonished by her capacity to evolve. I believe that she greatly needed what the analytic process was able to offer her, and that this encounter within the framework of the affective proximity of the transferential bond took place at an optimal moment for her possibilities of achieving psychic structuring. Could it be the magic of her achievements that she is showing? Or could it perhaps be the "magical powers" of an omnipotent fantasy of denial of loss? With a mixture of magic and pain, we got through our farewell.

References

Bonifacino, N. (2014). Avatares del devenir sujeto [Avatars of becoming a subject]. Clínica psicoanalítica con tempranos [Psychoanalytic clinic with young children]. *Uruguaya Psicoanál Journal, 119,* 57–73.

Bonifacino, N. (2017). De la precariedad psíquica a la subjetivación [From psychic precariousness to subjectivation]. Proceso analítico de una niña pequeña [The analytical process of a young girl]. *Madrid Psychoanál Journal, 81,* 265–293.

Freud, S. (1905). *Three essays on the theory of sexuality* (Vol. VII, Standard ed.). London: Hogarth Press, pp. 123–246.

Freud, S. (1907). *Creative writers and daydreaming* (Vol. IX, Standard ed.). London: Hogarth Press, pp. 141–154.

Freud, S. (1908). *Infantile sexuality* (Vol. VII, Standard ed.). London: Hogarth Press, pp. 173–206.

Klein, M. (1940a [1987]). *The importance of symbol formation in the development of the ego. Selected works* (Vol. 5). New York: The Free Press, pp. 95–114.

Klein, M. (1940b [1989]). *Mourning and its relation to manic depressive states. Complete works* (Vol. 2). Barcelona: Paidós, pp. 279–301.

Krauss, N. (2005). *The history of love.* New York: W.W. Norton & Company.

Laplanche, J. (1989 [1997]). New foundations for psychoanalysis: The original seduction. The theory of seduction and the problem of the other. *International Journal of Psychoanalysis, 78,* 653–666.

Winnicott, D. (1945 [1981]). Primitive emotional development. In *Writings on paediatrics and psychoanalysis* (Spanish ed.). Barcelona: Laia.

Winnicott, D. (1958 [1981]). The capacity to be alone. In *The maturational process [and the facilitating environment]* (Spanish ed.). Barcelona: Laia.

Winnicott, D. (1960 [1981]). Ego distortion in terms of true and false self. In *The maturational process* (Spanish ed.). Barcelona: Laia, pp. 169–184.

Winnicott, D. (1962 [1981]). Ego integration in child development. In *The maturational process* (Spanish ed.). Barcelona: Laia, pp. 65–74.

Winnicott, D. (1967 [1979]). Mirror-role of mother and family in child development. In *Realidad y juego* (Spanish ed.). Barcelona: Gedisa.

2 Psychoanalysis of young children with autism spectrum disorders. An adaptation of technique in the approach to three cases[1]

1 *Previous versions of this paper have been published in Revista Uruguaya de Psicoanálisis* (Bonifacino, 2014) *and* International Journal of Psychoanalysis (Bonifacino, 2023).

At present, the therapeutic approach for young children with autism spectrum disorder is a major challenge for child psychoanalysis.

These patients place us in a special clinical and metapsychological terrain with its own characteristics and call our technique into question. What tools do we have for working in situations where speech has not yet acquired a communicative value? How can we intervene when an experiential subject has still not been constituted? How can psychoanalysis benefit these patients?

The purpose of this communication is to show an adaptation of technique in the treatment of three children who came to my practice between the ages of two and three with a diagnosis of autism spectrum disorder.

In this context, there were certain elements that in the affective proximity of the transference bond which encouraged the child's openness to representational world and a progressive psychic structuring and subjectivation. These elements were the analyst's active search for an encounter with the child, the non-verbal exchanges between analyst and patient, and the characteristics of the interpretations.

As this is a clinical communication, it is not my intention to focus on a historical perspective of the psychoanalytic approach to severe childhood disorders. Nor do I intend to address the question of the aetiology of these clinical pictures, nor dispute the diagnosis with which these patients have been referred to me. In my experience, and beyond the three cases I am going to present later, each of the children with severe disorders who came to my practice had a history of sustained communication failures in their early relationships, regardless of the causes that generated this situation, which were always complex and multifactorial. Likewise, Bush de Ahumada and Ahumada (2015) indicate that all the cases of children with

DOI: 10.4324/9781032614823-4

autism they have treated showed traumatic incidences in the form of early cumulative traumas, which dislocated or distorted the affective "primary dialogue" (Spitz, 1964) between the infant and its mother (p. 20).

According to Tustin (1986), these authors base their technique on the analyst's "receptivity" and "quality of attention" and argue that the analyst must wait for signs of the child's spontaneity in order to attempt an interpretation and achieve fleeting "moments of contact" (p. 38). Thus, they oppose transference interpretation from the outset, considering the child's recognition of the analyst's presence to be a necessary condition in order for a transference relationship to begin to evolve. Bush de Ahumada and Ahumada (2015) propose that, since such children place the analyst's mind in a prolonged state of "silence" (p. 33), we cannot speak of countertransference in these situations. In the same vein, Meltzer (1995) states that with such patients, the mind (of the analyst) does not work, as there is very little material to observe (Meltzer, 1995, pp. 48–49). Cecchi (2013), on the other hand, points out that the analyst must tolerate the feelings of deep anguish, loneliness and hopelessness that these patients convey and proposes an expectant and active attitude, waiting for any sign that allows understanding and generation of accurate interpretations (p. 62), and convey to the child what is happening to him/her. Like Cecchi, Alvarez (2012) is against a neutral and containing psychoanalytic stance (p. 1).

There is also divergence on whether or not to incorporate work with parents into the child's process. Bush de Ahumada and Ahumada (2015) do not see any need for this. They meet with parents only occasionally, in the belief that this relieves the pressure on them. In contrast, for Joyce (2010) the analyst's own work with the parents is a condition for the child's treatment. Greenspan (2001) focuses his approach on the early relationship between the child and the parents, and Cecchi (2013) proposes family therapy alongside the child's treatment.

In the work with the patients I mention next, the analyst's active positioning, the vicissitudes within the transference-countertransference dyad and the proximity of the parents to the child's treatment and evolution proved to be essential elements of the analytic process. Interspersed with the clinical material I shall present some hypotheses and aspects of the technique that favoured communication and the encounter with these patients. Finally, I shall present a series of structuring progressions which, in each of these processes and in a unique way, showed the evolution of these children.

The original state

> The key word . . . is dependence. Human infants cannot start to be except under certain conditions. . . . Infants come into being differently according to whether the conditions are favourable or unfavourable.
>
> (Winnicott, 1960b, p. 43)

Within the psychoanalytic literature, various authors who start out from very different approaches arrive at the same point in supposing that the presence of the object (the other) is a primordial factor for the constitution of the subject (Winnicott, Laplanche, Roussillon, Bleichmar, Fonagy and Target, among others), postulating that the encounter with the other lays the bases for subjectivation. According to Roussillon (2015), just as a subject does not conceive itself as a physical being, neither does it form itself psychically. Highlighting the incidence of the other in the formation of the subject, he adds that "our psychic organisation depends not only on events and how we have signified them, but also on the dialectic between our psychic processes and the echoes necessarily received from the environment" (2015, p. 185). Freud also said in 1921: "In the individual's mental life someone else is invariably involved, as a model, as an object, as a helper" (p. 69).

Based on the clinical perception of the difficulty that the children with whom we are dealing had in grasping the presence of the other (the analyst), which reveals a lack of resources to establish an encounter, the following question arises: if the subject is formed in relation to the other, then what is there originally?

According to Freud (1926), the original state is one of helplessness. The child remains fundamentally given over to original helplessness. Laplanche argues on the basis of Freud's contributions that it "necessarily relies on the other both to satisfy its needs and to avert danger" (1989, p. 105). Taking up this notion, this author adds that there is originally "a state of helpless being . . . the state of a being who, left to himself, is incapable of helping himself; he then needs the help of others". At first "the excitement bubbling up from within overflows", he adds, "the mother quickly learns to recognise screams, movements, disorganised agitation as a call for help" (Laplanche, 1989, p. 101).

This idea immediately conjures up clinical pictures for me. The manifestations that Laplanche mentions, so primary and anchored in the body – *screams, movements, disordered agitation* – those expressions that appear as raw discharges, which need to be recognised by another, semanticised from a maternal function as a "cry for help", are aspects which have been at the forefront of the work with the patients to whom I am referring. I believe that the overflow of intense and confusing drives, which are triggered in a chaotic way in the form of a disorderly and uncontained agitation, persisted in these children as an element that expressed helplessness in the face of the impact of *the excitation coming from within* or, in other words, the drive:

> *Tiago is almost 3 years old. The neuropaediatrician has diagnosed him with pervasive developmental disorder. He rushes into the office for the first time, without looking at me. He walks back and forth in an uncontrolled manner, occasionally bumping into the armchairs that are in his path. He gets up awkwardly and hurries on unsteadily. When running, his arms and legs*

seem to move independently, without any harmony or coordination. At one point, he picks up a little human figure made of modelling clay that instantly falls apart due to his abrupt and forceful handling.

I point out that he, too, suddenly feels helpless in the face of a very great force that he feels within himself.

Tiago unexpectedly picks up a marker and makes very strong strokes on the blackboard, gritting his teeth and showing significant tension in his hand and facial expression; for an instant his face is distorted. His line tends to repeatedly to collide with the edge of the blackboard, which acts as a limit to his motor discharge.

I tell him that he is showing me his need for a firm framework which can contain that great force that he feels inside himself and that won't allow him to stop.

When the analyst's words are aimed at pointing out and providing a framework for experiences, it is interesting to note Winnicott's conceptualisation of "holding", which emphasises maternal emotional proximity as a necessary condition for subjectivation. According to this author, the "holding" refers not only to the physical act of sustaining the infant, but that it also "includes the management of experiences that are inherent in existence" and drive satisfaction, "which are determined by the awareness and the empathy of the mother" (1960a, p. 44). Winnicott adds that during infancy, which he takes to mean the preverbal, pre-symbolic period, the dominance of the "id" and the possibility of its incorporation into the "ego" will depend on maternal care (1960a).

In these complex insights into the early psyche, I see a starting point for very divergent theorisations, referring to two levels of experience that are intimately linked and converge in the process of subjectivation. I refer, on the one hand, to primary intersubjective experiences and, on the other hand, to the observational level of early interactions. A further complication of early experiences, as Laplanche (1989) puts it, is that the other protagonist of the original situation is an adult who cannot be conceived without taking into account her unconscious dimension. Alongside clinical practice, I shall consider the contributions made by both perspectives to reflect upon certain interventions by the analyst which, in the context of the affective proximity of the transferential bond, encouraged a progression towards symbolisation and subjectivation in the children in question.

Object activity and symbolisation

Based on Winnicott's (1945) assertion that the conditions that enable subjectivity are strongly rooted in holding, Roussillon highlights the mode of presence of the object within this framework, insofar as the activity of the object is revealed as a key element to promote primary processes of symbolisation in the subject (2015).

This conceptualisation of object activity – the active participation of the analyst – has been developed by Schkolnik (2007) as an important contribution to the analysis of neurotic patients with split elements, which refer to representational deficits caused by failures in the primary processes of symbolisation. In such situations, the author suggests the need for the analyst, as the object that enables symbolisation, to offer the patient representations that promote paths of psychic linkage, and therefore of containment, in the face of the overflow of the split – the drive – that is not symbolised. In this sense, the primary representations would give rise to the original repression, understood to be an association of representations, which would be formed as the founding element of the psychic apparatus.

The proposal of an analyst who offers representations of aspects that the patient is unable to symbolise by him or herself is an interesting perspective to think about certain technical resources which I recognise in the work with the infants to whom I refer. As seen at the start of Matilde's analytical process (Chapter 1), in the face of precarious functioning, words can be offered to represent those things which have not yet become organised in the child through personal experience. This would take on an organising value for the inner world and facilitate ways of working on building a psychic space and a psychic framework. Moreover, on certain occasions the words offered by the analyst would respond to the patient's expectation to have their perceptual world organised and thus rendered identifiable and sharable.

Javier, 2 years and 8 months old, does not speak. The neuropaediatrician has ruled out an organic disorder. His parents say he flits around the house aimlessly. They see that he is overwrought and worry that he bumps into things and carries on walking on as if he doesn't feel anything. In the first interview, Javier's father carried him in and encouraged him to go and play with the equipment on the floor. Sitting opposite him, I notice that he shyly touches some of the elements.

Showing willingness to generate some contact, I name them as he touches them: "The paper, the little cars, the wool. You want to get to know these things here," I say to him. "We are going to play together so that you feel better."

From then on, Javier starts to look me in the eye, and although the gesture is not sustained, I still find it encouraging. He then actively points to the markers one by one, and I name the different colours. I accompany his gestures with words. At times he tries to speak but makes unrecognisable sounds which neither the father nor I can understand. However, at a certain point, when he is taking animals out of a basket and I am naming them, we hear him say, still with difficulty, "We play." The father and I look at each other in surprise: the word, the verb, has emerged in an encounter with another person, in a libidinal bond.

Then Javier goes to the window and looks out. I go with him. We look at the view together; he points, and I offer him words that enable him to identify his perception of the world.

However, when verbal language has not yet become established as a means of communication nor to create a representational world, I wonder how much the child really grasps the meaning of words. In this respect, I find interesting the connotation that Target attributes to the analyst's word in reference to borderline patients, whose representational world is also precarious. In such situations, Target considers interpretations to form part of a dialogue that is for the most part conducted non-verbally or in some sense pre-verbally. The patient, much like an infant with a parental figure, hears the words but does not so much understand their meaning as the attitude behind them, the intention and the emotional tonality. The words are sounds that inform the infant about how the other feels in relation to her (Target, 2013). In the same vein, and with reference to patients with psychosomatic symptoms, in whom affect is not expressed in terms of words or symbols, Killingmo (2006) argues that rather than the semantic content of the interpretations, it is the very intonation and sound quality of the analyst's voice that conveys the emotional meaning of the experiences to the patient.

Up to this point I have focused on the analyst's word, a fundamental instrument of our technique that we recognise to be of indispensable value for generating meaning and enabling paths of representation and psychic association. However, in child psychoanalysis, the word is not the only register of communication. The child analyst's *free-floating attention* is not just paid to the patient's verbal communication but also to what the child does and what happens in the encounter, whether or not in a playful register. Particularly in the work with the patients to whom I am referring, in the absence of the child's communicative language, gestures and non-verbal communication acquired greater significance. The first sessions with Matilde, described in Chapter 1, illustrate these aspects.

Non-verbal exchanges

> What does the baby see when he or she looks at the mother's face? I am suggesting that, ordinarily, what the baby sees is himself or herself. In other words, the mother is looking at the baby and what she looks like is related to what she sees there.
>
> (Winnicott, 1967, p. 148)

In order to reflect on the scope of the non-verbal elements of communication in working with the patients to whom I refer, I shall draw on conceptualisations that come from observations of early mother-baby interactions. Numerous psychoanalytic authors identify primary elements of dyadic communication, which encourage the baby's self-perception, as well as the recognition and regulation of emotions, among other aspects. The acquisition of these elements is distorted in the children in this study.

In this context, rhythm, mutuality and synchrony in the back and forth of interaction are identified as organising principles of the infant's psychic life (Stern, 1985; Benjamin, 2002). Underlying these elements is an affective attunement that mother and baby achieve together on the basis of mutual influence and adaptation, which requires the activity of both protagonists (Stern, 1985; Beebe et al., 2016). At the clinical level, various fragments of the work with Matilde illustrated these aspects, for example, the shared song (Chapter 1).

From another perspective, it has also been pointed out that, in daily dyadic communication, the mother naturally adds certain resources of her own to her gestures. These are accompanied by words that designate emotions, desires and intentions that she perceives in the baby and which generate a key scenario to give rise to certain intersubjective processes. In these situations, the mother's vocal and facial expressions spontaneously acquire peculiar characteristics that are identified in an affected or high-pitched tone of voice, marked gestures and an exaggerated facial expression or "maximisation" in her own face of the expression of affection that she attributes to the baby (Gergely and Watson, 1996). These manifestations have been considered as natural "mirroring" phenomena, in which the maternal face is offered as a representation of the emotional state of the baby that it cannot yet identify and feel as its own. This is a first form of symbolisation, which arises in the context of early bonds based on empathy and identification of the mother with the baby, and which would be essential to enable phenomena of greater complexity in the incipient psyche.

These contributions present an interesting way of thinking about certain communications between the analyst and patient that go beyond words, and which, in the precarious functioning of the children in the present study, took on an interpretative value. In the context of the affective closeness of the transference relationship, the analyst's marked facial and gestural expressions that highlighted the child's emotional experience, as well as the different emotions that the analyst conveyed in his vocal tone, became resources that arose spontaneously in the encounter, and which also conveyed meaning. In this way, in the work with the patients to whom I am referring, from elementary forms of communication, the analytical intervention in a non-verbal register was generating a framework of "mirroring" of the experiences, which enabled the patient to get in touch with them and to recognise them as their own.

Structuring movements

The child psychoanalyst works on the boundaries of or from within child psychosis, but always on the borders of it and confronted with a diversity of movements of passage, real moments of structuring of the psychic apparatus.

(Bleichmar, 1984, p. 220)

I shall now present some significant moments in the work with each of the children to whom I have referred. These accounts describe a progression from elementary to more elaborate psychic processes, and together they illustrate the construction of a psychic organisation and structure that was gaining in richness and complexity. In the context of each patient's analytic process, and as structuring events, these episodes marked the inauguration of new forms of functioning, while at the same time they showed enriched symbol use.

In the situations to which I shall refer, the appropriation of new resources was gradually configuring an internal organisation and enabling psychic work by containing drives by linking representations and creating buffers and distinctions. Alongside these progressions, words flowed freely as a means of expression, generating a certain openness and mobility of meaning, and the iterative "I" was used in language to represent the psychic subject.

Javier and the capacity for association

After a year and a half of analysis, at almost 4 years of age, Javier talks about himself in the first person in language that has emerged in the context of a playful and libidinal bond. Even so, his vocalisations are still poor and disorganised, or limited to set phrases, with little original content. Difficulties in pronunciation prompted a speech therapy consultation, and he was diagnosed with a language disorder. Javier was showing the functioning of a younger child, and I was concerned about his development.

From the first year of treatment onwards, we worked without the presence of his parents in the practice, and in general he was very willing to come to his three weekly sessions. On one occasion, in the context of a game we were sharing, Javier identified a fruit in an image and named it, saying, "pineapple." He then looked at me and added, "The pineapple doesn't prick." This verbalisation catches my attention, because I notice that it implies the association of the object with an experience, and this is something new in Javier's speech. "Sometimes it does prick," I tell him, holding his gaze. "You have to be careful."

Continuing the dialogue and as if seeking reaffirmation from me, he looks at me again and asks, "Do mosquitoes prick?"

"Of course, and pineapples also sometimes prick. Maybe that reminded you that mosquitoes prick and bite."

"You have to put band-aids on," adds Javier.

In this brief dialogue, Javier showed an incipient capacity to associate his own representations, experiences and sensations and to express them verbally. All of these progressions were showing a certain symbolic development and implied a certain representational mesh, and that psychic functioning was becoming more complex. From then on, during the sessions he used some of his own words that connoted his experiences. In terms of transference, I saw this process momentum as ushering in of a new form of communication, which means I have to make less effort to make contact. Words began to gain ground, whether through questions, short dialogues, songs and rhymes that we shared, or to accompany play. The new psychic organisation also offered new possibilities for intervention.

Tiago and the father's place

Six months into a process of three weekly sessions and based on a favourable evolution, both the treating psychiatrist and neuropaediatrician indicate that their former diagnosis of pervasive developmental disorder no longer applied. In the framework of the analytical relationship, Tiago had been integrating language as a way of transmitting his ideas and had been appropriating his body through his experiences. However, he still had a strong need for an organising and holding framework in the face of what he perceived as a difficulty in containing his impulses and a threat that they could not be contained. In this sense, his discourse increasingly contained an insistent appeal to the father figure.

At a certain point, a year and a half into the analysis and at just over 4 years old, Tiago's father was away on business. The boy was able to reflectively express his sadness, saying, "I don't like Dad to leave. I like him to be with us. But he doesn't like to leave either, he's going to work." At this point in the process, even with his difficulties Tiago can get in touch with his feelings within the analytical framework without becoming disorganised, and he can use language adequately. At the same time, he is also showing signs of major psychic development in that he is also capable of recognising and expressing the emotions of the other.

At this stage, the father was an identifying referent, taking on a valued place, and enabled the child a display of phallic power that he rehearsed through fighting games, personifying superheroes, who confronted what he called "the baddies".

Tiago has come a long way. He can perceive himself as a subject, discriminate symbolic places and place himself in a masculine generational plot. The father figure would henceforth be positioned as an oedipal rival, opening the way to structuring conflicts.

Matilde: new expressions of old complaints

Finally, in relation to Matilde, the sequence presented in Chapter 1, starting with the session titled "Making the girl", shows a gradual process of subjectivation and psychic structuring, which enabled the child to experience the typical vicissitudes of infantile neurosis. Matilde's analysis took three and a half years, during two of which our sessions took place three times a week. When analysis ended, the girl was well into her first year of school.

A few years after the process was complete, her mother came to see me. She said that Matilde was still at the same school, to very high standards, and that, although she is considered to be an intelligent child, her performance is uneven. I note with concern that the changes in the family environment had not been as sustained or supportive as I would have liked. When I receive Matilde, who has just turned nine, I find her to be an affectionate and communicative child who has noticeably structured an infantile neurosis. "My old friend Nahir!" she says in greeting. There is a deep bond of affection between us. During a series of encounters, she tells me horror stories, which she says frighten her. In one of these, there is a woman who kills children. "The story has a moral for parents," she says, "for them to be with their children. It's a horrible story, because it's like having your heart empty." I sense that Matilde suffers from loneliness. Even so, she now has resources which allow her to express her devastation, her desire to have a mother who is affectively closer, and her anxieties, without becoming disorganised or overwhelmed by them. In a series of sessions, she repeatedly suggests we play a game in which we take turns to make a portrait of each other, looking at each other closely in order not to omit any details of the face to be drawn. Could it be a new and more elaborate version of the search for a gaze and a face that, like a mirror, allows her to recognise herself?

I find that Matilde's way of being in this new encounter highlights the value of the analytical bond, and it moves me. She has come for a reunion, and she expresses this in her greeting. The richness of her emotional expressions and verbal communication contrasts sharply with my memory of that little girl from the initial sessions. She has achieved a dynamic psychic organisation with symbolic resources that allow her to convey, through fantasies, her distressingly deep loneliness, her affects and conflicts. But her helplessness is no longer devastating, and the experience of the analytical bond seems to linger, resonating within her as a face in which she can look at herself, find herself, recognise herself and feel seen, found, and recognised.

Modifications of technique: conclusion and discussion

According to psychoanalytic theorisations on the beginnings of psychic life, the constitution of the subject takes place in the encounter with the other and in intersubjective terms. The process of subjectivation, that is, of coming to perceive oneself as the subject of experiences, with the representation of one's own body and with the possibility of using language enunciated in the first person (I), also implies the acquisition and deployment of ego functions, that is, language, motor skills, attention, the ability to think, among others. All these functions are impaired in young children with autistic spectrum disorders.

The three patients to whom I have referred presented with excess excitement that found an outlet in the body, without any link to words or other symbolic representations. This functioning revealed that the underlying motive for the anxiety and defences that these children displayed were not a response to psychic conflict. Rather, what was at stake was the acquisition of an experience of identity, that is to say, of subjective existence. On the basis of these elements, in the approach to these children the primary task was to generate the conditions to make room for the complex dynamics at play in the construction of the psyche and on the way towards symbolisation and subjectivity. The affective closeness of the transference bond – a psychoanalytic element by nature – was a key scenario, insofar as it was presented to the child as a new opportunity for encounter and subjectivation.

In the three cases presented, *"receptivity"* and *"quality of attention"* as elements of technique (Bush de Ahumada and Ahumada, 2015; Tustin, 1986) were inseparable from the active participation of the analyst in the search for an encounter with the child. I took the patient's limited manifestations through the lack of impulse control, subtle gestures, sketches, inhibitions, decontextualised words, fragmented sentences or changes in body posture as a potential starting point for an encounter, giving it a meaning and a communicative value from the countertransferential grasp. In this way, the analytic intervention was aimed at generating for the child an experience of being looked at and recognised as a subject of experiences.

Along the same lines, *"receptivity"* and *"quality of attention"* also implied *free-floating attention* which, given the precariousness of the child's psychic functioning and the lack of representational language, was directed towards a non-verbal register. Furthermore, this non-verbal dimension also spontaneously arose in me as a technical resource to represent the patient's emotional states. Thus, my gestures, my facial expressions and different tones of voice which went along with the child's emotional experience and my words had a communicative effect. Throughout the clinical material I have presented, I was interested in pointing out the gradual changes in the patients' functioning as they incorporated a representational register that gave rise to a subjective experience of themselves. As Killingmo (2006) argues, the representation of affect and the representation of the self come from the same symbolic matrix and take place gradually throughout a process of ego-differentiation, which takes place within the framework of an intersubjective relationship.

From this perspective, in the analysis of these patients the transference relationship would not be considered in the sense of repetition, as classically described by Freud in his articles on technique (1912, 1914). On the contrary, in these situations the therapeutic relationship provided the child with a novel space in the encounter with another, generating experiences in which each member of the analytic dyad contributed something that was both unique and authentic (Stern et al., 1998). In other words, the analyst, with his emotional availability, and with his active modality in the encounter with the child, presented himself as a new object, which enabled the patient to enter into a symbolic dimension which led to subjectivation.

One aspect that merits special consideration concerns the interpretation or not of the destructive impulses with which these children presented. As shown in the clinical material, at the beginning of the process I did not ascribe any intentionality or aggression to these impulses towards the other or the analytic space, although this could have been an option. On the other hand, the countertransferential grasp of the experience of fragility, loneliness and disconnection that these children conveyed led me to consider these manifestations to be overflows of excitation (Laplanche, 1989) and an expression of the lack of ego resources for the physical containment and psychic processing of uncontrolled impulses, which subjected the child to experiences of helplessness and fragmentation. In my understanding, interpreting these impulses as having an aggressive or destructive intentionality would require greater ego integration on the part of the child, which was gradually being achieved throughout the analytic process, giving rise to interpretations of aggressiveness – and also of sexuality – in terms of unconscious desires and conflicts. On the other hand, in the situation of non-integration (Winnicott, 1962) that predominated in these patients at the beginning of the treatment, I understood that the possible interpretation of the overflow of impulses with an aggressive or destructive intentionality could generate greater inhibitions in the child, sharpening their disconnection and further weakening their incipient psychism.

In summary, in the cases presented, modifications in the analyst's technique contributed to significant internal changes in each of the patients, both in communication with the analyst and in the child's communication with themselves and with the most significant others in their family and social context.

An important element in the evolution of the previously mentioned cases, which however was only roughly portrayed throughout the clinical material, concerns the proximity of the parents in relation to the child's analytical process. I believe that this is an area in which multiple aspects converge, such as the characteristics and availability of the parents, their transferential aspects towards the child's analyst, and even the young child's own need to be accompanied by a parent at the beginning of the analytic process. Given these complexities, this issue deserves to be analysed in depth and on a case-by-case basis, which is beyond the scope and limits of this chapter. However, in general terms and given the child's physical and emotional dependence on his or her parents, I believe they are decisive not only for the permanence and regularity of the treatment but also to generate certain conditions in the family dynamic itself that allow the patient's gradual evolution to be actively supported. In my experience, it was very important to have regular interviews with the parents, which enabled me to transmit aspects of the child's experiences and functioning that they were unable to understand, in order to promote greater sensitivity towards the patient's problems and suffering. I understand that, beyond the difficulties, limitations and resistance on the part of the parents, these meetings tended to favour a transference scenario that benefited the work with the child and also the patient's relationship with his or her parents. In some of the cases referred to, the mobilisation that these interviews aroused in some parents led to them to seek out their own therapeutic space.

Finally, it should be noted that, as mentioned previously, the adaptation of the technique I have illustrated in the three cases presented had positive effects on the evolution and outcome of treatment. This has also been confirmed in my clinical experience with other young children who shared the same functional characteristics. However, clinical communications and systematic research of various kinds will allow further investigation of the impact of the described modifications of technique on the positive evolution of psychoanalytic treatments of young children with autism spectrum disorder.

References

Alvarez, A. (2012). *The thinking heart: Three levels of psychoanalytic therapy with disturbed children*. London: Routledge.

Beebe, B., Messinger, D., Bahrick, L. E., Margolis, A., Buck, K. A. and Chen, H. (2016, April). A systems view of mother-infant face-to-face communication. *Developmental Psychology, 52*(4), 556–571. https://doi.org/10.1037/a0040085; Epub: 15 February 2016; PMID: 26882118; PMCID: PMC4808406.

Benjamin, J. (2002). The rhythm of recognition. *Comments on the work of Louis Sander. Psychoanalytic Dialogues, 12*(1), 43–53.

Bleichmar, S. (1984 [2008]). *En los orígenes del sujeto psíquico [On the origins of the psychic subject]*. Buenos Aires: Paidós.

Bonifacino, N. (2014). Avatares del devenir sujeto [Avatars of becoming a subject]. Clínica psicoanalítica con tempranos [Psychoanalytic clinic with young children]. *Uruguaya Psicoanál Journal, 119*, 57–73.

Bonifacino, N. (2017). De la precariedad psíquica a la subjetivación [From psychic precariousness to subjectivation]. Proceso analítico de una niña pequeña [The analytical process of a young girl]. *Madrid Psicoanál Journal, 81*, 265–293.

Bonifacino, N. (2023). Psychoanalysis of young children with autism spectrum disorders. An adaptation of technique in the approach to three cases. *The International Journal of Psychoanalysis, 104*(1), 23–45. https://doi.org/10.1080/00207578.2022.2149403

Bush de Ahumada, L. and Ahumada, J. (2015). Contacting a 19-month-old mute autistic girl: A clinical narrative. *The International Journal of Psychoanalysis, 96*(1), 11–38.

Cecchi, V. (2013). Algunas consideraciones acerca del autismo. [Some considerations about autism]. In *Autism clinics: Controversies. Controversies in Child and Adolescent Psychoanalysis. Journal*, (13), 59–64. Buenos Aires: Psychoanal. Association.

Freud, S. (1912 [1976]). *On the dynamics of transference. Complete works* (Vol. XII, Spanish ed.). Buenos Aires: Amorrortu.

Freud, S. (1914 [1976]). *Remembering, repeating and working through (Further recommendations on the technique of psycho-analysis II). Complete works* (Vol. XII, Spanish ed.). Buenos Aires: Amorrortu.

Freud, S. (1921 [1976]). *Mass psychology and analysis of the self. Complete works* (Vol. XIX, Spanish ed.). Buenos Aires: Amorrortu.

Freud, S. (1926 [1976]). *Inhibition, symptoms and anxiety. Complete works* (Vol. XX, Spanish ed.). Buenos Aires: Amorrortu.

Gergely, G. and Watson, J. S. (1996). The social biofeedback theory of parental affect-mirroring: The development of emotional self-awareness and self-control in infancy. *The International Journal of Psychoanalysis, 77*(6), 1181–1212.

Greenspan, S. (2001). The affect diathesis hypothesis: The role of emotions in the core deficit in autism and in the development of intelligence and social skills. *Journal of Developmental and Learning Disorders, 5*(1), 1–44.

Joyce, A. (2010). Discussion of Jorge L Ahumada and Luisa Busch de Ahumada's paper. In M.Leuzinger-Bohleber, J.Canestri and M.Target (Eds.). *Early development and its disturbances*. London: Karnac, pp. 175–183.

Killingmo, B. (2006). A plea for affirmation relating to states of unmentalised affects. *The Scandinavian Psychoanalytic Review, 29*(1), 13–21. https://doi.org/10.1080/01 062301.2006.10592775.

Laplanche, J. (1989 [2001]). *New foundations for psychoanalysis. La seducción originaria [Original seduction]* (Spanish ed.). Buenos Aires: Amorrortu.

Meltzer, D. (1995 [2002]). *Psychoanalytic work with children and adults: Meltzer in Barcelona*. London: Karnac, p. 49.

Roussillon, R. (2015). La fonction symbolisante de l'objet. [The symbolizing function]. *Jornal de Psicanálise, 48*(89), 257–286. Recuperado em 21 de junho de 2024, de http://pepsic.bvsalud.org/scielo.php?script=sci_arttext&pid=S0103-583520150 0200020&lng=pt&tlng=fr.

Schkolnik, F. (2007). El trabajo de simbolización Un puente entre la práctica psicoanalítica y la metapsicología [Symbolisation work A bridge between psychoanalytic practice and metapsychology]. *Revista Uruguaya de Psicoanálisis, 104*.

Spitz, R. (1964). The derailment of dialogue: Stimulus overload, action cycles, and the completion gradient. *Journal of the American Psychoanalytic Association, 12*, 752–775.

Stern, D. (1985). *El Mundo Interpersonal del Infante [The interpersonal world of the infant]*. Buenos Aires: Paidós.

Stern, D., Sander, L., Nahum, J., Harrison, A., Lyons-Ruth, K., Morgan, A., Bruschweiler-Stern, N. and Tronick, E. (1998, October). Non-interpretive mechanisms in psychoanalytic therapy. The 'something more' than interpretation. The process of change study group. *The International Journal of Psycho-Analysis, 79* (Pt 5), 903–921. PMID: 9871830.

Target, M. (2013). *Regulation of affect. In 48th IPA congress*. Prague.

Tustin, F. (1986). Psychotherapy with psychogenic autistic states. In Autistic barriers in neurotic patients. New Haven, CT: Yale University Press, pp. 286–308.

Winnicott, D. (1945 [1981]). Primitive emotional development. In *Writings on paediatrics and psychoanalysis* (Spanish ed.). Barcelona: Laia.

Winnicott, D. (1960a [1981]). Ego distortion in terms of true and false self. In *The maturational process* (Spanish ed.). Barcelona: Laia, pp. 169–184.

Winnicott, D. (1960b [1981]). Theory of the parent-infant relationship. In *The maturational process [and the facilitating environment]* (Spanish ed.). Barcelona: Laia.

Winnicott, D. (1962 [1981]). Ego integration in child development. In *The maturational process* (Spanish ed.). Barcelona: Laia, pp. 65–74.

Winnicott, D. (1967 [1979]). Mirror-role of mother and family in child development. In *Realidad y juego* (Spanish ed.). Barcelona: Gedisa.

3 Clinical intervention with a 15-month-old toddler at risk of autism and her mother

Juanita is brought to the clinic by her mother when she is 15 months old. She has recently been diagnosed with being at risk of autism and presents noticeable difficulties in relating to others. Her face is expressionless, and she avoids eye contact. She has no verbal expression.

The dynamics of the dyad reveal important maternal fragilities and ambivalences that hinder the possibility of separation and differentiation. In this context, Juanita's disconnection seems to arise as a reaction to a bond that, rather than providing a framework of containment for early arousal, exposes the toddler to the intrusive presence of the mother's body and breast and thus to an excess of arousal, with a disturbing effect.

The first two clinical encounters with Juanita and her mother are described and analysed, in which the analyst's interventions promoted novel, playful and pleasurable experiences in the dyad that enabled the child to enter a symbolic and subjective dimension, with access to the word as representation.

The approach was based on contributions from observational studies of the mother-infant dyad interaction, psychotherapeutic approaches to early bonds and psychoanalytic theories of the early psyche.

First encounter

15-month-old Juanita arrives at the clinic in her mother's arms. Her face is expressionless. She turns her head from side to side in an automatic gesture without looking anywhere and doesn't seem to register my presence. I find her appearance striking. The mother is feebly holding her, and when Juanita moves, they both become unsteady. I offer the mother a seat, where she sits with the toddler in her arms.

I sit opposite them, near a low table on which I set out some play equipment. I greet Juanita by name, but she shows no sign of responding. She continues to move her head automatically and to avoid eye contact. In the face of this lack of response, Juanita's mother tells me that she does not respond to her name, that she also does not look at her and that she is very worried about this. She says that a few weeks ago she had taken her to a

DOI: 10.4324/9781032614823-5

specialist clinic, where, on the basis of the techniques used, they diagnosed Juanita as being at risk of autism.

In a renewed attempt to establish contact, I take a toy horse from the table, turn to the toddler and say,

A: "Juanita, I brought these toys for you. I wonder if you like them? Do you know the little horses?"
     From her mother's arms, the toddler, who until then had her back to me, turns and looks at me expectantly for a few moments. I think this reaction was probably motivated by the high-pitched tone of voice I spontaneously used when addressing her. Although her face remains expressionless, I find her response a little encouraging. To encourage further contact, I then offer her the toy horse I am holding in my hand. However, she twists in her mother's arms, turning her back to me again.

A: "Let's see. Do you like this chicken better? Cluck-cluck-cluck," I say slowly and with a playful intonation, while offering her this other toy. Juanita turns to me again, looks at the toy chicken, takes it from my hand and drops it, without looking at me.

A: "Oops! It fell down! Where has the little chicken gone?" I ask in an enthusiastic tone, building some anticipation.

I pick the toy up from the floor and offer it to her again. She picks it up again and drops it. A sequence thus takes place in which Juanita looks at the toy, takes it from my hand and drops it, looking at the floor. Then, in an expectant voice, I ask, "Let's see, where did the chicken go?" and finally I pick it up, saying in surprise, "Here it is!", and offering it to her again. This sequence is repeated several times under the mother's close scrutiny.

At a certain point, Juanita turns her back to me and rubs her face against her mother's body, who quickly puts her nipple in her mouth, saying that the child feels sleepy.

Note I. Here-gone.
   The way Juanita and her mother present concerns me greatly. The mother conveys fragility and bewilderment, and the child shows no initiative or willingness to interact. She seems to be absent. Given these characteristics, I consider that I need to take the initiative in trying to establish contact. This is my intention when I look at her, talk to her and offer her the toy. Juanita responds to my initiative by reacting a little. She looks up at me briefly, turns to me from her mother's arms and takes the chicken from my hand to drop it.
   Then, in the manner of the "fort-da" ["gone-there"] which Freud described in his observations of his grandson playing with a cotton reel (Freud, 1920) and in an elementary exchange with the toy hen, a sequence is generated between the two of us in which Juanita drops the object – making it disappear – and then it reappears, and I show it to her. This activity stages a

very significant and structuring experience of the early psyche, which Juan-
ita thereby acquires: presence-absence is a fundamental binary opposition
that mobilises the process towards symbolisation. The question arises as to
whether she expected from the outset that I would offer her the toy again, or
whether she simply dropped it due to her own disconnectedness or lack of
interest? I am inclined to believe the second option. Perhaps it was the active
and creative positioning of an other-analyst in a symbolising object func-
tion (Roussillon, 2015) that was enabling the child towards an original and
novel experience. As Winnicott puts it (in Playing and Reality, a Theoretical
Statement, 1967, p. 54): "where playing is not possible then the work done
by the therapist is directed towards bringing the patient from a state of not
being able to play into a state of being able to play".

However, the mother's subsequent initiative in pulling the toddler towards
herself, and more precisely to her breast, interferes with and obstructs the
precarious resources that Juanita is developing for processing the separation
and the absence of the object, which ultimately refers to the separation from
the primary object: the mother. In this sense, the mother's intrusive gesture
of quickly inserting her nipple into Juanita's mouth seems to indicate strong
maternal resistance to a certain openness on the part of the toddler to estab-
lish contact with the other-analyst, such as occurs on this occasion through
the toy.

I perceive a mother who comes to the consultation genuinely concerned
and seeking help, but who also presents significant difficulties in making
space for a third party in the bond with her daughter. Given my impression
of the situation and the feeling of insecurity and fragility conveyed by the
mother, I intervene from a descriptive register, as will be seen below, pointing
out Juanita's abilities while recognising the mother's role and her mater-
nal identity. As has been argued, in the approach to early bonds, maternal
sensitivity is an element that adds complexity for the analyst's intervention
(Stern, 1995). The situation becomes even more complex when sustained
dyadic mismatches expose the child to risk in early emotional development
and early psychic functioning (Winnicott, 1945), as is the case between
Juanita and her mother.

A: "But you saw that she was playing," I say to the mother: "She threw the
    toy and I gave it to her, and she threw it again hoping that I would give
    it back to her. This is a very important game because Juanita is showing
    us in this way that she is processing the experience of separating from
    you and knowing that she will find you again, just as she separates
    from the toy and takes it again and again."

    The mother looks at me, listening attentively. She then detaches Juan-
    ita from her breast, looks at her and hugs her. She tells me that they live
    alone and that she has been separated from the child's father for more
    than a year. She adds that since the two of them are alone in the house
    for several hours a day, she has a large television on to entertain Juanita.

M: "And she doesn't talk at all, maybe because the television is on all day. I thought she liked that," she reflects.

A: "But!" I say to the toddler with higher pitched, slower intonation, and she responds to my gaze. "Mummy thought you liked watching television, Juanita, but it seems to me that you like to be looked at and talked to, don't you?"

"Ah . . . ah . . . ah . . ." she says, looking at me and making sounds for the first time. She then turns on the spot and with a certain excitement presses her mouth against her mother's cheek, who hugs her again.

A: "You are showing us that you like to chat," I say, talking to Juanita in an enthusiastic tone, "and also that you love Mummy very much."

M: "Is she talking?" asks her mother, looking at her daughter affectionately. However, to my surprise she immediately pulls the child to her breast and again places her nipple in Juanita's mouth. The child rather awkwardly latches on for a brief moment and then moves away from the breast.

A: "She wants to be with you because you are her mother, and she loves you very much, and she wants to continue being your baby. But not being quite so close to you helps her to grow up. Sharing a toy, singing to her, showing her a picture book. Where does she sleep?" I ask.

M: "Oh, no! No! Don't tell me that! Don't tell me to take her out! She sleeps with me in my bed, so if she wakes up at night I breastfeed her and she carries on sleeping. She just has a little bit more, hardly any for a little while each time, all night long."

I tell the mother that it would help Juanita to have her own bed and to sleep in her own room.

As we say goodbye and I have closed the door, I can hear the mother singing to her daughter as they wait for the lift.

Note II. Sketches of verbal expression.

Within the analytical framework, Juanita can begin to establish eye contact and express herself in simple, elementary vocalisations directed at a third party. However, in the face of the toddler's new movement towards differentiation and relating to the analyst, the mother again responds intrusively by appropriating Juanita's body and imposing her nipple in her mouth. The child's initiative to use her own voice to express herself ("ah . . . ah . . . ah . . .") and access speech is thus blocked by maternal interference, which leaves no room for the symbolic dimension.

Some hypotheses about the dynamic development between the mother and daughter occur to me. On the one hand, I notice that, despite her difficulties, and to the extent that she does not see me as an intrusive presence, Juanita is demonstrating that she has a certain capacity to relate, for example, by looking at me several times or by emitting certain sounds. So could her disconnection and gaze avoidance be an expression of a primary defence (Fraiberg, 1982; Salomonsson, 2016; Viaux-Savelon et al., 2022) *that arises as a reaction to a mother-daughter bond which, instead of providing containment for early arousal, exposes Juanita to an intrusive presence of the maternal body and breast, and thus to an excess of arousal that impacts on the incipient psyche, disturbing it? (Benjamin and Atlas, 2014).*

And in this context, how can I introduce a third party who can enable Juanita to differentiate and symbolise without becoming an intrusive presence myself which causes the mother to respond by rejecting the intervention that she and her daughter need? Due to this question, and noticing the mother's need to keep a distance, I suggest that they do not return for another week, and not before as would have been desirable, due to the problematic dynamics of the dyad and their negative consequences on Juanita's early psyche.

Second encounter

On the day we agreed to meet, Juanita's mother called and said it would be difficult to bring the child to the consultation. We then arranged to hold the second session a few days later.

When I open the door, Juanita is in her mother's arms. She looks at me, turns away and cries, repeating this sequence a few times.

The mother becomes anxious and insecure. She sits with the child in her arms and says she doesn't know why she gets like this, "because she was fine, and she didn't use to be like this . . ."

A: "And since when have you seen her like this?" I ask.

M: "and . . . since she knows where we are going, before she was more prone to . . ."

A: "Of course," I say, "but she's older now, and she notices when she's with people she doesn't know, and that makes her feel insecure. She wants to meet other people, which is why she looks at me from time to time, but she's also a bit frightened."

As Juanita hears my voice speaking calmly and slowly, she turns in her mother's arms to look at me.

A: "Isn't that right, Juanita?" I say, looking at her. "You feel safe and cared for with Mummy."

She turns back towards her mother again and rests her open mouth on her cheek.

The mother is very touched and says, "oh, the little darling", hugging her. She then sits the child on her knees, facing me. I notice that Juanita maintains her gaze on me. I perceive that when I acknowledge in words how important it is for Juanita to feel safe and cared for by her mother, the latter feels greatly relieved. She is then also more inclined to allow the toddler to interact with me.

However, Juanita's mother interrupts Juanita's gaze as she is looking at me, quickly offering her the toy hen on the table. The child cries, rejects it and turns away. "Don't you want it?" her mother says, visibly affected by the child's response. "But last time you played with the little chicken," she adds, referring to our previous session.

She then takes other toys from the table, offering them to her daughter, but Juanita refuses these, too, and cries again.

I find the misunderstanding I perceive in the dyad distressing. The mother insists on her offer and expresses frustration and distress at the toddler's continued rejection and crying. I sense that although intervening at this point might help Juanita to calm down, it might also make the mother feel inadequate or disparaged, which could increase her fragility. I therefore refrain from acting or speaking and wait.

Then the mother picks up a book from the table and shows it to Juanita. "She likes picture books," she says.

The child initially rejects the book by turning her head away but then turns around and begins to look carefully. She spontaneously points to some pictures as her mother turns the pages.

"What a nice book," says the mother. "We could get one like it to keep at home, Juanita." And looking at me, she adds, "She has a picture book that she likes very much, and I've brought it. Can I show it to you?"

A: "Of course," I say, encouraging her. And then, turning to the child, I add, "It's good that Mummy brought the picture book, Juanita. Mummy knows you very well, and she knows what you like!"

Her mother takes the book out of a bag and offers it to Juanita, who is interested in it and turns the pages herself. This time, it is the mother who points to pictures while briefly describing what they can see together. Juanita looks at her mother, looks at the book and briefly vocalises after listening to her mother.

A: "You like looking at the book with Mummy," I tell her. "You are reading it together!"

The mother smiles in relief. "Yes, she really likes it when we read books."

Note III. Initiative and communicative intent.

In this second meeting, there is still resistance on the part of the mother. She seeks help and shows concern, but at the same time keeps me at a distance.

At first, perhaps sensing the mother's contradictory messages, Juanita is staging the difficulty of including me as a third party in her gestures of refusal. In the therapeutic approach to early bonding, the words addressed to the child – in this case concerning her fears and insecurities – are also heard by the mother and may acquire a certain resonance for her in relation to her own unconscious aspects (Lebovici, 1988; Cramer and Palacio Espasa, 1993; Stern, 1995). Then, feeling acknowledged by me in her maternal role and valued in the preference the toddler shows for her, the mother can turn Juanita round on her lap to face me, thus allowing her contact with me.

However, the mother's ambivalence asserts itself, and in an intrusive move she offers Juanita different toys in quick succession, each of which the child refuses in turn. Despite this misunderstanding in the dyad, I value Juanita's active rejection of her mother's intrusive attitude. I notice that instead of withdrawal or avoidant disengagement, the toddler begins to manifest more vital impulses and reactions (Guedeney, 2007).

Then, after twisting and turning quite a bit, Juanita becomes interested in the book that her mother takes from the table, and a very significant scene takes place. By spontaneously pointing and inviting the mother to look at pictures in the book that arouse her interest, the child displays a gesture that has been attributed an important diagnostic value in early socio-emotional development. It is a gesture of shared attention, which implies a communicative intention, together with a move towards differentiation and recognition of the other. That is, by pointing to the pages of the book with her finger, Juanita is actively and spontaneously showing her initiative in getting her mother to look at something that is unfamiliar to both of them and that they can share together.

In response, and noticing Juanita's interest, the mother says to her, "What a nice book, we could get one like it to keep at home." Her message is ambiguous. Does the mother recognise that a third party-analyst is able to offer something attractive-valuable which interests Juanita, and then proposes to get a similar one because of its implied value? Or on the other hand, would "having one like it at home" be a way of not needing and negating the presence of a third party for both Juanita and her mother? Given the vulnerability I perceive in the mother, I do not interpret her ambivalence. I understand that pointing this out might seem intrusive, untimely or even feel like an attack on her ability to provide care and attention to the child, further affecting her image of herself as a mother.

In this vein, however, when the mother then offers Juanita the picture book she has brought for her, and they look at it together, I do point out that the mother knows the child well and how much Juanita enjoys sharing this activity together. Taking into account the specifics of the transference dynamic that unfolds in the support of mother-baby dyads, a fundamental element of which is the mother's sensitivity, the act of recognising and pointing out the mother's capacities, as well as the value for the baby of what the mother offers her, tends to foster a higher sense of worth in the mother (Stern, 1995). At the same time, not perceiving me as a disparaging figure may encourage her to be more accepting of my presence and interventions.

After a few minutes of looking at the book with her mother, Juanita loses interest and shifts uncomfortably in her lap. Sensing this situation, I ask the mother if the child is already starting to walk. Smiling and proud, she says that she is, adding that she can also climb all over the place. At the same time, she takes Juanita off her lap and helps her stand on the floor. The toddler spontaneously climbs nimbly onto the couch next to her. She clambers up and down repeatedly, enjoying her movements.

A: I tell her, "You can do all that, Juanita! Just like Mummy said!"
       At a certain point, Juanita looks at her from the edge of the couch, stretches out her little arms and throws herself towards her mother, who holds onto her. Juanita shows relief, and enjoys being held by her mother.
A: "Wow, how strong Mummy is! How she held onto you! You liked it!" I add.
       She climbs back onto the couch.
A: "I think you're going back," I say in an animated and expectant voice. Then, I describe and accompany Juanita's gestures with my words and the tone of my voice, while she stretches out her little arms again towards her mother: "One, two and . . . three!!" says the mother enthusiastically, adding to my expectant words, and also enjoying this activity with Juanita. When the toddler rushes towards her, she holds her tightly and hugs her with a smile on her face.
       A lovely encounter occurs between them. For the first time, I notice a hint of a smile on Juanita's face. She is enjoying the encounter with her mother and the expectation of being held by her.
       "Yes, she likes to play," says the mother, happy, and seeing Juanita smile.
       The toddler continues to show subtle changes in facial expression. She arches her eyebrows slightly in surprise and continues with faint smiles as she seeks and holds more eye contact with the mother's gaze, and with me as well.
       After repeating this game a few times, on her own initiative Juanita sits on her mother's lap, facing me, and looks at me expectantly. I also look at her and smile, making a comment of some kind. Then, I take the toy horse from the table and make the sound of hoof beats.
       The mother repeats the sounds I make and also the tone of my voice, adding, "the horsie".
       ssJuanita looks at me attentively. I notice that she looks at my lips and slowly imitates the movement of my mouth, until, very quietly, she imitates the sound as well.
A: "You're making the sound the horsie makes," I say to her.
       She climbs down from her mother's lap and stands, holding on to the table and the armchair.
M: "I'm worried that she's not talking yet," says the mother. "How can I help her?"
A: "You saw that she is looking at us more and trying to relate, and that is very important to be able to start talking. Do you talk to her?"
M: "Yes, but maybe too much. Since I want her to talk, I insist."

A: "Well, it's important that you realise this. Juanita is showing signs that she is going to talk. Maybe you could talk to her, without insisting, while you are feeding her, or at bath time. Does she like to spend time in the bath?"

M. "Yes, and she has a duck that she plays with," replies the mother, with a smile.

Suddenly, we hear Juanita's voice saying "cua", and we both look at her in surprise.

A: "How attentive you are, Juanita! And you show Mummy that you do talk. You made the sound the duck makes in your bath."

I tell the mother that these words of Juanita's are very important because they show us that she is listening to us carefully and that she understands and is participating in our conversation.

M: "Really?" says the mother, visibly moved. "I am very touched by what you say, because I was very worried about her." She is upset. "I thought I had harmed her, because she didn't look at me. She doesn't call me Mummy," she adds, crying and very distressed.

Juanita, standing next to her mother's armchair, approaches her and gently places her mouth on her cheek. The mother also hugs her gently. The toddler then spontaneously stands up and walks towards a French window behind the armchair, her back to her mother. She stands there holding on to the glass with her little hands. It is already night, and the window acts like a mirror. Suddenly, she begins to make sounds, looking at her image in the glass. She makes long syllables, with different intonations: "ooooohhh-hhhh . . . eaaaaaaahh . . . eeeeehhhhh". She seems to be listening to herself and playing with her voice.

I show the mother that Juanita is starting to talk, that she imitated the horse's voice, that she said "cua-cua" when she heard her mother mention the duck in the bath and that maybe when we meet again, she will already be chatting and saying "mama".

Concluding remarks and reflections. Opening up towards a symbolic dimension.

After my acknowledgement of the toddler's enjoyment of sharing the book with her mother, and in response to my question about Juanita's ability to walk, the mother takes her down from her lap in a careful gesture of detachment. A number of significant events then took place. Firstly, the toddler shows significant mastery of her movements, and climbs spontaneously and with agility, enjoying her physical display. In contrast to the automatic head gestures that took place in the first encounter, this time Juanita shows that her body belongs to her, and that she can use it intentionally. To paraphrase Winnicott (1945), the – incipient – psyche inhabited the soma.

Secondly, stimulated by the analyst's words and her expectant tone of voice, the toddler and her mother become active protagonists in a playful activity which they both enjoy and which again recreates the experience of separation and the prospect of being reunited. Climbing on the couch, Juanita looks at her mother and throws herself into her arms, expecting to be held, while the mother's gestures and words encourage Juanita's sense of expectation, and she responds by holding her affectionately at the moment when the toddler is waiting for her. Mother and daughter live and feel a playful and pleasurable experience together (Winnicott, 169, 1971). From another perspective, it is also an experience of affective attunement (Tronick, 2007), a fundamental element on the way to achieving subjectivity. Moreover, the mother, who is emotionally involved in this activity, joins in with the analyst's expectant words, enthusiastically adding the number "three" – the third one – which is also introduced as a representation from the playful space.

Juanita ends this activity by spontaneously sitting on her mother's lap and facing me. She looks at me expectantly, available for the relationship. It is then that she looks and imitates the movement of my lips when I make the sound of the horse's hooves, and then she imitates the sound too, in a barely audible voice. Thus, a series of expressions take place that form a universal sequence in language acquisition (Bruner, 1977): looking at the other's lips, imitating movement and imitating the sound of the voice. In this sense, it is a key moment when Juanita spontaneously says "cua-cua" when she hears her mother's reference to the toy duck. It shows that she is attentive to what is happening around her, involved in the relationship, understands the words and is actively participating in the dialogue. Moreover, by alluding to the toy duck through the sound that represents it, Juanita is proclaiming her entry into the world of representational language, in other words into a symbolic universe.

The mother is moved and relieved by the connotation I attribute to the toddler's words and her ability to develop, perhaps then being able to express painful feelings such as anguish, fragility and a negative perception of herself as a mother, afraid she has harmed Juanita. Experiences that refer to unconscious aspects (Laplanche, 1989) connected with her own history, which are reactivated and interfere in the dyad bond (Cramer, 1989; Fraiberg et al., 1975). The toddler senses her mother's distress and goes towards her affectionately, but she also has the initiative to disengage herself from her mother's embrace.

In the final sequence, Juanita is leaning against the window when she discovers her own image in the mirror, which she looks at and speaks to with some surprise and glee. In other words, in a highly significant event in the early psyche, Juanita discovers herself in the mirror. The perception of her body as being her own, which was expressed in the fluidity, mastery and enjoyment of her movements as she spontaneously climbed up and down the couch and onto her mother's lap, is now transferred to the image. That is to say, to a new register that implies a new dimension of representation.

To conclude, I believe that during these two initial encounters, the analyst's presence and active participation, which was both sought after and negated in function of maternal ambivalence and resistances, introduced novel elements into the dynamics of the dyad. These encouraged a process of separation and differentiation, enabling Juanita to acquire an incipient representation of herself and elementary outlines of a communicative language, thus opening up towards a shared and symbolic world.

References

Benjamin, J. and Atlas, G. (2014). The 'too muchness' of excitement: Sexuality in light of excess, attachment and affect regulation. *IJP Open – Open Peer Review and Debate*, 1, 1–35. [+ *The International Journal of Psychoanalysis*, (1), 39–63, 2015].

Bruner, J. (1977). Early social interaction and language acquisition. In H. R. Schaffer (Ed.). *Studies in mother-infant interaction*. New York: Academic Press, pp. 271–289.

Cramer, B. (1989). *De profesión bebé [Baby by profession]*. Barcelona: Uranus.

Cramer, B. and Palacio Espasa, F. (1993). *La pratique des psychoterapies meres-bébés: Étude clinique et technique*. Paris: Presses Universitaires de France.

Fraiberg, S. (1982). Pathological defences in infancy. *The Psychoanalytic Quarterly*, 51(4), 612–635. PMID: 6758010.

Fraiberg, S., Adelson, E. and Schapito, V. (1975). Ghosts in the nursery: A psychoanalytic approach to the problems of impaired infant-mother relationships. *Journal of the American Academy of Child & Adolescent Psychiatry*, 14(3), 387–421.

Freud, S. (1920). Beyond the pleasure principle. In J. Strachey (Ed.). (1966) *Standard Edition of the complete works of Sigmund Freud* (Vol. XVIII). London: Hogarth.

Guedeney, A. (2007). Withdrawal behaviour and depression in infancy. *Infant Mental Health Journal*, 28(4), 393–408.

Laplanche, J. (1989 [1997]). New foundations for psychoanalysis: The original seduction. The theory of seduction and the problem of the other. *International Journal of Psychoanalysis*, 78, 653–666.

Lebovici, S. (1988). *El Lactante, su madre y el psicoanalista: [The infant, its mother and the psychoanalyst: Early interactions]*. Buenos Aires: Hogarth Press.

Roussillon, R. (2015). La fonction symbolisante de l'objet. [The symbolizing function]. *Jornal de Psicanálise*, 48(89), 257–286. Recuperado em 21 de junho de 2024, de http://pepsic.bvsalud.org/scielo.php?script=sci_arttext&pid=S0103-5835201 5000200020&lng=pt&tlng=fr.

Salomonsson, B. (2016). Infantile defences in parent-infant psychotherapy: The example of gaze avoidance. *The International Journal of Psychoanalysis*, 97, 65–88.

Stern, D. (1995). *The motherhood constellation: A unified view of parent-infant psychotherapy*. New York: Basic Books, Hachette Group.

Tronick, E. Z. (2007). Interactive mismatch and repair: Challenges to the coping infant. In E. Z. Tronick (Ed.). *The neurobehavioral and social-emotional development of infants and children*. New York: Norton & Co, pp. 155–163.

Viaux-Savelon, S., Guedeney, A. and Deprez, A. (2022). Infant social withdrawal behavior: A key for adaptation in the phase of relational adversity. *Frontiers in Psychology*, 13, 809309. https://doi.org/10.3389/fpsyg.2022.809309.

Winnicott, D. (1945). Chapter XII: Primitive emotional development. In *Through paediatrics to psychoanalysis: Collected papers*. New York: Brunner-Routledge, pp. 145–156.

Winnicott, D. (1967). Chapter 3: Playing, a theoretical statement. In *Playing and reality*. London: Tavistock Publications, pp. 38–52.

Winnicott, D. (1969 [1991]). The mother-infant experience of mutuality. In D. Winnicott (Ed.). *The collected works of D. W. Winnicott*. London; New York: Routledge, pp. 131–140.

Winnicott, D. (1971). Chapter 38: The mirror-role of mother and family in child development. In *Playing and reality*. London: Tavistock Publications, pp. 211–218.

4 Technology and the early psyche. The impact of video technology on two young children with severe disorders[1]

1 *A previous version of this paper was published in Revista Uruguaya de Psicoanálisis (2017) No. 125. (Bonifacino, 2017)*

Technology has long since become incorporated into our daily lives. Children are born and grow up in environments saturated with technological elements, and their access to them is favoured from a very early age. Moreover, the very attractiveness of the image on screens – from the television, tablet, mobile phones and computer, with their diversity of colours, sounds and movements – coupled with offerings that are promoted as being aimed at children of different ages, have turned technological media into a resource that parents frequently use to entertain and soothe their young children (Hutton, 2013; Paudel et al., 2016).

At the same time, excessive exposure of children to screens is a matter of concern for a number of child health care disciplines (Engelhardt et al., 2013; Mazurek and Engelhardt, 2013; Radesky and Christakis, 2016; Duch et al., 2013). For example, recognised paediatric associations and government health departments in different regions recommend that parents limit their children's screen time and even that they should not use screens until the age of two. They also warn of difficulties that may arise in early childhood when the virtual world tends to displace the child's interest in bonding with others and suggest that young children's screen exposure should always take place in the company of an adult, and never alone (Argentina Society of Paediatrics (2020), American Academy of Pediatrics, Australian Government Department of Health (2024), among others).

Child psychoanalysis is no stranger to this subject. The impact of technology on children's psychic functioning has reached our practices and raises new questions and challenges. In modern day clinical practice, we observe children of different ages who are at risk of becoming hooked on various technological devices. When this fixation is very marked and occurs in young children with severe disorders, it is interesting to reflect on its impact on early psychic functioning and on the process of subjectivation.

This chapter aims to address this issue on the basis of two children who were a few months over the age of 2 when they came to my practice. Both

DOI: 10.4324/9781032614823-6

had been previously diagnosed as severely disturbed by neuropaediatricians and child psychiatrists. One of the children had a diagnosis of autistic spectrum disorder, while the other was diagnosed with pervasive developmental disorder. Fixation on videos was present in both situations.

In the first case, we shall consider a sequence that takes place during the initial meetings with the patient and his parents, and in which certain elements of the video that captured the child's attention and tended to isolate him from his environment are incorporated into the analytical framework in a playful way, taking up a transitional place (Winnicott, 1951/1981) that opens the way to a creative, subjective and symbolic universe.

In contrast, the second set of material offers elements for thinking about the impact of technology in terms of overstimulation and over-excitation, along with the consequences that these experiences imply for early psychic functioning and the process of subjectivation.

From screen fixation to playful activity

First meetings with the child and parents

Fabian's parents come for a consultation when the child is 2 and a half years old. They were concerned. They say that Fabian does not speak, does not look them in the eyes, that "he seems to be in a world of his own", and that he "is always glued to the video". "The video is the only thing he is interested in, and he asks for it insistently," they add. "If we don't let him watch it, he starts running around and we can't stop him. It's like an addiction. He's mesmerised by the screen, and sometimes he falls asleep."

As for Fabian's early life, they say that there had been several changes of caregiver during his first year, and that when he was 13 months old, the person who took care of him while his parents were working left, at which point they decided to send him to preschool. They recognise that this stage was very distressing for the boy, who could not stop crying. They add that this period coincided with a business trip that the father went on for several months.

Fabian arrives at our first meeting in his mother's arms. She places him on the floor, near some baskets of toys. With an abrupt gesture, the boy quickly and completely overturns them. Everything lies scattered about. He immediately stands up and moves to a table which has some play equipment on it. There, he picks up and puts down each of the toys at random. With the intention of trying to make contact, I approach him and name the objects he is picking up. I look him in the eye and tell him that it seems to me that he wants to get to know things in this place, which is new to him. But Fabian doesn't look at me or give any sign of registering my presence. Instead, he begins to quickly pace about from one side of the consulting room to the other, overwhelmed by anxiety.

As his parents had explained, Fabian does not look people in the eye. He does not seek the gaze of the other. Not even his mother's. There is no encounter with a maternal gaze that can libidinise and act as a mirror and containing framework for the intensity of early experiences (see Chap. II. Winnicott, 1967). I understand that Fabian's difficulties reveal a history of early bonding failures or discontinuities. In other words, a history of major misunderstandings that have significantly marked his psychic functioning (see Chap. II. Laplanche, 1989).

At a certain point, and still without looking at her, Fabian brings a toy to his mother, who is still in the consulting room. I consider this search for contact to be a very significant gesture. I tell him that he seems to want to share things with Mummy, although I doubt the child can grasp my meaning. However, this message is also addressed to his mother (see Chap. III). Fabian then picks up a toy cup and places a spoon inside. "You're playing at cooking!" I add in an enthusiastic tone. I perceive the child's gesture as a slight move towards a symbolic dimension, and I point this out to the mother as a positive aspect.

Then Fabian picks up a two-wheeled trolley from among the scattered toys. He cannot get it to move on his own. At the same time, he picks up a small car with his other hand and, with difficulty, tries to put them together. Sitting down on the floor next to him, I tell him that I think he wants to hook them together but that it's difficult to do so, and he might need help. I hold these toys together with him and show him how to connect them. I notice that Fabian accepts my intervention, looks at me fleetingly for the first time and leaves the toys in my hand while he watches carefully as I hook them up, as he intended. I put them together and give them back to him. He then rolls the trolley and the car together on the ground. I think of his need to "hook" himself into a bond that helps him function, but I don't mention this. Fabian has not made any sounds as yet and makes practically no gestures. At times, he is disconnected, his gaze wandering into nothingness.

A few days later, he visits again. He arrives at this second session with his father. On entering the consulting room, he repeatedly throws and scatters toys and also throws small lumps of modelling clay on the floor. I understand that, in terms of Winnicott (1945), he is thus manifesting an experience of non-integration (Chapter 1, pp. 4, 6). I tell him to show me the scattering, which is perhaps how he feels himself, without any restraint or containment. Fabian then takes some bits of modelling clay from the floor and sticks them on a piece of paper. Following his initiative, I help him to make them stick on the paper, pressing the chunks of modelling clay down once he has placed them while commenting on what I am doing. The boy watches me, and then he gives me other bits of modelling clay and also watches the way I stick them together. I intentionally make a gesture of exaggerated effort as I press each time. At times, Fabian looks me fleetingly in the eye and smiles faintly. I notice that he is showing some gratification and that he enjoys these brief exchanges. Libidinal aspects begin to flow. I then tell him that I think he is enjoying doing this together and that maybe he also needs to be glued like the modelling clay: "glued to Mummy, to Daddy, in order to grow up".

The child then takes a marker and draws lines on a piece of paper with such uncontrolled force that it makes a hole. I perceive that, in contrast to the joining – the gluing – there has been a rupture. I find myself thinking about the impact the interruptions and discontinuity of his constant loss of caregivers and his father's absence may have had on him, but I keep this impression to myself and say nothing.

Then Fabian gets the trolley hooked up to the car that we attached last time and goes back to scattering bits of modelling clay. I pick up one of these little bits from the ground, mould a little ball and offer it to him. He takes it in his hand, briefly looks at me and smiles. Then he himself puts a small piece of modelling clay in my hand and squeezes forcefully, imitating the way I had squashed the modelling clay onto the paper. I understand that he wants to attach it to my hand. A certain possibility of a bond is being established.

I will now focus on the issue at hand. Through a sequence that begins in the initial sessions, certain elements of the video that focused Fabian's attention and isolated him from his environment are incorporated into the analytical framework in a playful way and acquire for the child a condition of dynamism and transitionality (Winnicott, 1951/1981) that enables him to move towards creative and symbolic movements, with favourable effects on the process of subjectivation.

Presence-absence

In the third session, Fabian spontaneously picks up a marker and practices making strong strokes on the whiteboard. When there is no more room, his father wipes the whiteboard, and the child starts drawing lines again. After doing this several more times, Fabian himself erases the lines. "You make them appear and disappear when you want them to," I tell him. I see this as a very significant movement, which like Freud's *fort-da* (Freud, 1920) recreates the presence-absence alternation, with a structuring value for the early psyche.

Fabian repeats this activity during subsequent sessions, which are three times a week. On one occasion, fearing a continuation of the repetitive action, on my own initiative I pick up a marker and, telling him what I am going to do, draw something that I think might be close to what the child is experiencing (see Chap. II).

"Let's see, do you like this?" I ask him, drawing a little car.

Fabian looks at what I'm doing, waits for me to finish and then vigorously erases it. "You didn't like it," I say with an expression and tone of exaggerated regret (see Chap. II).

Fabian stops, looks at me and pauses with what I take to be an air of expectancy. A sequence then takes place in which I draw while telling him what I am going to do, he looks attentively at the image that appears on the whiteboard, then quickly and somewhat mischievously erases it and waits for me to draw something else. He enjoys this activity.

At some point, his father, who is watching these exchanges closely, follows my initiative, fetching a marker and saying he is going to draw something he knows Fabian likes very much.

"It's Kevin's boat, in the cartoon which Fabian always asks to watch and gets very angry when we turn off the video," he adds.

Fabian is surprised by the image of the pirate ship on the whiteboard. I ask some questions, which encourage the father to add details to the drawing, explaining as he does so: this is the treasure chest, the anchor etc. Fabian watches attentively and with interest. He erases some of the details that he does not seem to like and also points out certain parts of the completed drawing of the ship, where the father realises some other object is placed, which he then also adds: the ship's sail, the rudder etc. I accompany this sequence with descriptive interventions, along with others that are aimed at libidinising the father-son bond, highlighting how well the father knows Fabian and how much he knows about what he likes.

In subsequent sessions, Fabian runs in, goes directly to the whiteboard and gives his father a marker, wanting to repeat this activity and participating in it actively and with great interest. I point out his initiatives, his invitation to his father and ask questions that support other details in the drawing and generate new encounters between father and son. Little by little, the exchanges about the ship are enriched with new elements, and the main character of the video, Kevin himself, who is a pirate child, becomes gradually incorporated into the repertoire drawn by the father.

Later, at the request of Fabian or his father, some toys from the play equipment are added to the scene on the whiteboard. Among these, there is a little doll representing Kevin, which Fabian places in different parts of the drawn boat while looking at his father and me expectantly. I accompany the boy's initiatives by describing the actions of the character depending on where he places him. For example, the little Kevin doll at the rudder is steering the boat, or he is spying land when Fabian places him atop the mast. The flat space of the whiteboard is thus gradually transformed into a playground, giving rise to varied and novel developments.

Recognising oneself in the other

In a later session, Fabian tries to stick bits of modelling clay on a sheet of paper, but the material is hard and does not stick the way he wants it to. I tell him that we have to "warm it up" to be able to play, and taking it in my hands, I soften it and form a little ball that I place in front of him on the table. I shape another piece of modelling clay into a small cylinder. Fabian looks at me expectantly. "Here's a little ball that's softer to play with, and here's a little snake," I tell him. However, he quickly picks up the cylinder of modelling clay, runs to the doll representing Kevin, and places one end of the cylinder in the doll's hand. He picks up the Kevin doll and shows it to me, looking at me.

"Is it like a sword?" I ask, frankly surprised by the child's creativity in this initiative. The father, also surprised, confirms that Kevin has a sword. Fabian then moves the arm of the doll, making the modelling clay sword move. He seems happy.

"What a good idea!" I say to him. "You made Kevin's sword!" He briefly looks at me and smiles. He then picks up the modelling clay cylinder himself and moves it back and forth, as he had done before with the doll. "Now you've got the sword! Like Kevin!" I say, as I watch him play. He smiles again.

I consider this scene to be a paradigmatic example of certain movements that take place in working with young children who present difficulties in the process of subjectivation. That is to say, just like the hard, cold lump of modelling clay that Fabian was unable to use, which I held in my hands to warm it up so it could be moulded, that which is cold and affectively distant becomes warm in the affective proximity of the transference bond, and that which is hard, fixed and static becomes malleable and transformable, taking on the outlines of a symbolic universe, in which the object is invested with potential meanings.

The richness of Fabian's creative act is also evidenced by the implied representations relating to a body image and the possibility of identifying with a human figure and recognising oneself in the other.

As we say goodbye, Fabian runs to the door with his fist clenched tightly. In it, I see he has the little doll holding the modelling clay sword. For some time after, he will bring this character from home to the consulting room, where it will play a central role in various developments. Among these, one game later in the therapeutic process particularly stands out: Fabian hides the doll, and after repeatedly checking that I am looking for it and have found it, he himself hides in the same place, enjoying the expectation and confidence of being found.

Of course, there was still a long way to go in the relationship between Fabian and his parents. Be that as it may, I see these significant movements that occur within the analytical framework as giving the child the chance to acquire new resources which he can use to process experiences. In the material presented, a sequence is occurring in which Fabian is able to leave the rigidity of the video image that trapped and isolated him, to transition through the image created by his father in the drawing on the whiteboard and, finally, to create the sword out of modelling clay himself as an attribute of the character with whom he himself later identifies.

The question arises: what enabled the child to move from a place of being a passive "spectator", for whom, according to the parents, the video had an almost hypnotic effect, to "inhabiting" the character, recognising himself in the protagonist and using this as the starting point for creation? In other words: What are the conditions that enable the video image to become a transitional object for Fabian (Winnicott, 1951/1981) which allows for displacements that enrich the experience and inaugurate the creative space

(Pelento, cited by Bareiro, 2012). I shall try to approach these questions by drawing on contributions that come from the study of mother-baby dyad interactions, and early bonds and intersubjectivity.

Overstimulation and withdrawal

As Benjamin and Atlas (2014/2015) state, based on the concept that the constitution of the subject evolves intersubjectively (Stern, 1985), the mother-baby interaction gains relevance for clinical work. At the origin, Laplanche points out that "the excitement that comes from within overflows" (1989/2001, p. 101), and the conditions for the containment and processing of this are generated within the framework of a bond of affective attunement (Fonagy, 2002; Benjamin and Atlas, 2014/2015).

However, when there are repeated and persistent difficulties in the affective attunement of the dyad, instead of generating a containing framework for early experiences (Chapter 2, Winnicott, 1960), the presence of the mother is instead associated with disconcerting or overwhelming responses and becomes in itself a source of overstimulation and anxiety (Benjamin and Atlas, 2014/2015). This generates in the incipient subject primary defences of withdrawal, disconnection or flight from a bond (Brazelton et al., 1975; Guedeney, 1997) which, instead of being organising and structuring for early psychic functioning, become disruptive (Benjamin and Atlas, 2014/2015).

I consider these contributions to be a possible starting point for thinking about Fabian's strong fixation on the video. According to the parents' account, two contrasting images of the child emerge. On the one hand, the anxious running back and forth in agitation when he is not watching the video. This would seem to indicate difficulties in containing his impulses and his emotional experiences, which overflow without containment. On the other hand, as long as Fabian is in front of the screen, his excitement is calmed and soothed.

From this perspective, Fabian's fixation on the video could perhaps be seen as a refuge or disconnection from a relational framework to which the parents say he was exposed from a very young age, which involved repeated experiences of discontinuities and losses that had a disturbing effect on him.

At the same time, perhaps this disconnection in the video implies a kind of distancing from an inner world of emotional experiences which, due to their intensity, the precariousness of the early psyche's resources and the loneliness in confronting them, overwhelm his capacity for psychic processing, and are instead manifested as physical tension, in the action of running anxiously and aimlessly about?

Finally, a new aspect to consider concerns the stimuli emitted by the screen image itself. How do we think it impacts on the early psyche? Why does the video, with its mix of movement, sound and colour stimuli, have a calming effect on Fabian instead of generating greater excitement? That is to say, paradoxical though it may seem, why do more stimuli do not produce more excitement in the child, as might perhaps be expected?

In the context of early mother-infant dyad interactions, a natural resource has been identified that is brought into play in the infant from early life to regulate the impact of stimuli when they exceed the infant's processing capacity (Tronick, 1978; Guedeney, 1997). Faced with an excess of stimuli, the baby withdraws behind a kind of defensive barrier, which at the height of its expression induces a state of sleep.

I believe that something similar may underlie the calming effect which Fabian's parents say the video has on him. In such case, although the child's attachment to the screen could be seen as a means of "escape" from a relational environment with disturbing characteristics and from the intensity of emotions, the technological device itself also exposes Fabian to stimuli that could be overwhelming or excessive and which lead to "drowsiness" as a way of protecting against them.

Concerning excess and its impact on the early psyche

In order to expand on this aspect of the overstimulation or excessive stimulation that can result from screen exposure in young children, I am going to draw on a brief snippet of clinical material on Tiago, who came to the clinic when he was 2 years and 8 months old. This patient presented significant difficulties in functioning and had a diagnosis of pervasive developmental disorder (PDD). He had a recurring attraction to films, videos and, later, electronic games. In the setting of an analytical process of three weekly sessions, and as he was acquiring communicative language, at the age of 4 Tiago would insistently recount scenes from films he had repeatedly seen. The impact these scenes had on him was reflected in a progressive increase in anxiety, growing disorganisation of his speech and in automatic and tense movements of his limbs. The intensity of the stimuli exceeded his psychic capacity to contain and process them.

As the analysis progressed, he used graphic resources to repeatedly draw sequences from films and video games, in the form of screens. I understood these drawn narratives within the context of the repetition necessary for the elaboration (Freud, 1920) and processing of stimuli that impacted on the child's precarious psyche and overwhelmed his capacity to integrate them as subjective experiences.

During a phase of positive development, and at the age of 5, one day Tiago arrived at the session noticeably ill at ease and with marked signs of tension, which I had not seen in him for a long time. With considerable anxiety and at an accelerated pace, he tells me that he had been playing PlayStation, but that he can't use it anymore because the TV screen is broken.

"I broke it," he says, "because I'm stupid. I was playing on the Play-Station, and it was always playing that same music, tac, tac, tac, tac, tac,

tac, tac, tac, tac, tac, tac, tac, tac." He repeats the same tune insistently in a fast rhythm, which seems to me like the sound of hammering, his anguish increasing all the while. "I couldn't bear to listen to it any longer!" he added, raising his voice and bursting into tears, looking into my eyes and conveying intense helplessness. "And I threw it at the TV and it stopped! Because the TV screen broke! And now it can't be used anymore! It makes me hate everyone! That's how it makes me feel!"

This is the extent of the material to be shared. I realise that Tiago, having already acquired resources that allow him to give an account of his experiences, can express in words how "unbearable" or "uncontainable" he finds the excess of stimuli. The action of throwing the PlayStation at the television screen arises in the child as a desperate, extreme resource to put an end to the excitement and anxiety that the video game aroused in him and which he found he had insufficient psychological resources to contain. Moreover, in his brief account, Tiago alludes to what he thinks of the adults who do not protect him from the intensity of these experiences, and he expresses the hatred that his helplessness towards them generates in him.

Finally, I would like to suggest that access to technology probably does not have the same significance and implications for all children, perhaps not even the excessive use of technology. However, I tend to agree with Benjamin and Atlas (2014/2015) in saying that when there have been major difficulties in containing and processing early arousal – which, beyond its multiple causes, refers to difficulties in the affective attunement of the mother-baby dyad – then the non-contained, which Benjamin and Atlas refer to as "the excess" of early experiences, "probably leads to anxiety and inability to tolerate any tension, or aroused affect" (p. 54). And I would add that these are experiences which then acquire a disorganising value for psychic functioning, as can be observed in Tiago's material.

According to this perspective, a question I have about the fixation on video technology in these patients with early pathology is whether it should be seen as a cause or a consequence of these children's difficulties in establishing contact with and relating to others. In other words, in such cases is a screen fixation a cause or a consequence of the difficulties in the process of subjectivation?

I would say it is both. That is to say – as could be observed in Fabian's material – this fixation functions as a refuge or "disconnection" in the face of an early bond that fails to process arousal. At the same time, exposure to the screen itself becomes a source of stimuli which, without the presence of another to process them, can be overwhelming and cause the child to withdraw even further, accentuating his or her "disconnection".

In terms of Benjamin and Atlas (2014/2015), it could be argued that a screen fixation blocks invitations to the other, but it is this invitation or search for a bond that in the framework of severe pathologies of early childhood is blocked by the experience that all excitement, that is, all bodily and affective arousal, is dangerous and uncontainable in the relationship with the other.

Returning to clinical practice, to Fabian and the sword scene, I believe the affective proximity of the transferential bond – a fundamental part of the analytic process: the "living and feeling together" or "the mutuality of experience" in Winnicott's terms (1969/1991) – is where a new experience of containment and regulation of arousal and affects is generated for the child, which allows the transformation of arousal into communication and symbolic play.

References

American Academy of Pediatrics Family Media Use Plan. www.healthychildren. org/MediaUsePlan.

Argentina Society of Paediatrics, Comité Nacional de Crecimiento y Desarrollo, Subcomisión de Tecnologías de Información y Comunicación [National Growth and Development Committee, Sub-Commission on Information and Communication Technologies]. (2020). *Uso de Pantallas en tiempos del Coronavirus [Use of screens in times of coronavirus].* https://www.sap.org.ar/uploads/archivos/general/files_uso-pantallas-epocacovid_1589324474.pdf (Accessed 5 September 2021).

Australian Government Department of Health and Aged Care. Physycal activity and exercise for all Australians. For infant, toodlers and preschoolers (birth to 5 years). (2024). https: www.health.gov.au.

Bareiro, J. M. (2012). *Clínica del Uso del Objeto. La posición del analista en la obra de D. W. Winnicott [Object use clinic. The position of the analyst in the work of D. W. Winnicott].* Buenos Aires: Letra Viva.

Benjamin, J. and Atlas, G. (2014). The 'too muchness' of excitement: Sexuality in light of excess, attachment and affect regulation. *IJP Open – Open Peer Review and Debate, 1,* 1–35. [+ *The International Journal of Psychoanalysis*, (1), 39–63, 2015].

Bonifacino, N. (2017). De la imagen al juego. Tecnología y clínica con tempranoscon dificultades en la subjetivación. [From image to play. thecnology and clinic with infants with difficulties in their subjectivation process]. *Uruguaya Psicoanál Journal, 125,* 29–42.

Brazelton, T. B., Tronick, E., Adamson, L., Als, H. and Wise, S. (1975). Early mother-infant reciprocity. *Ciba Foundation Symposium, 33,* 137–154.

Department of Health. (2015). *Australia's physical activity and sedentary behaviour guidelines.* Australian Government. http://www.health.gov.au/internet/main/publishing.nsf/content/health-pubhlthstrateg-phys-act-guidelines#npa05.

Duch, H., Fisher, E. M., Ensari, I. and Harrington, A. (2013). Screen time use in children under 3 years old: A systematic review of correlates. *International Journal of Behavioral Nutrition and Physical Activity, 10,* 1–10.

Engelhardt, C. R., Mazurek, M. O. and Sohl, K. (2013, December). Media use and sleep among boys with autism spectrum disorder, ADHD, or typical development. *Pediatrics, 132*(6), 1081–1089. https://doi.org/10.1542/peds.2013-2066; Epub: 18 November 2013; PMID: 24249825.

Fonagy, P. (2002). *Affect regulation, mentalisation and the development of the self.* New York: Other Press.

Freud, S. (1920). Beyond the pleasure principle. In J. Strachey (Ed.). (1966) *Standard Edition of the complete works of Sigmund Freud* (Vol. XVIII). London: Hogarth.

Guedeney, A. (1997). From early withdrawal reaction to infant depression: A baby alone does exist. *Infant Mental Health Journal, 18*(4), 339–349.

Hutton, J. S. (2013). Baby unplugged. *Clinical Pediatrics, 52*(1), 62–65.

Laplanche, J. (1989 [1997]). New foundations for psychoanalysis: The original seduction. The theory of seduction and the problem of the other. *International Journal of Psychoanalysis, 78*, 653–666.

Mazurek, M. O. and Engelhardt, C. R. (2013, August). Video game use in boys with autism spectrum disorder, ADHD, or typical development. *Pediatrics, 132*(2), 260–266. https://doi.org/10.1542/peds.2012-3956; Epub: 29 July 2013; PMID: 23897915.

Paudel, S., Leavy, J. and Jancey, J. (2016). Correlates of mobile screen media use among children aged 0–8: protocol for a systematic review. *Systematic Reviews, 5*(1), 91.

Radesky, J. S. and Christakis, D. A. (2016, October). Increased screen time: Implications for early childhood development and behavior. *Pediatric Clinics of North America, 63*(5), 827–839. https://doi.org/10.1016/j.pcl.2016.06.006; PMID: 27565361.

Stern, D. (1985). *The interpersonal world of the infant: A view from psychoanalysis and developmental psychology*. New York, NY: Basic Books.

Tronick, E. (1978). The infant response to entrapment between contradictory messages in face-to-face interaction. *Journal of the American Academy of Child Psychiatry, 17*(1), 1–13.

Winnicott, D. (1945 [1981a]). Chapter XII: Primitive emotional development. In D. Winnicott (Ed.). *Through paediatrics to psychoanalysis: Collected papers*. New York: Brunner-Routledge, pp. 145–156.

Winnicott, D. (1951 [1981b]). Chapter 1: Transitional objects and transitional phenomena. In D. Winnicott (Ed.). *Playing and reality*. London; New York: Routledge, pp. 1–157.

Winnicott, D. (1967 [1979]). Chapter 38: The mirror role of mother and family in child development. In D. Winnicott (Ed.). *Playing and reality*. London: Tavistock, pp. 211–218.

Winnicott, D. (1969 [1991]). The mother-infant experience of mutuality. In D. Winnicott (Ed.). *The collected works of D. W. Winnicott*. London; New York: Routledge, pp. 131–140.

5 From repetition to novelty. The analyst's play as a creative resource in encounters with a child who has a serious disorder

This chapter presents a selection of the clinical material of a 5-year-old boy who came to the clinic at the age of 3 with a diagnosis of autistic spectrum disorder.

During the first two years of the analytic process, with sessions taking place twice a week, the patient showed gradual evolution. However, from a certain point onwards, he began to display a frankly confrontational mode in the sessions and marked oppositional defiance that also crept into his family and school life. This dynamic was sustained over many months, interfering with the child's growth and learning process.

In this case, I am not going to refer to the initial encounters with the patient and his parents. However, I am particularly interested in delving into this other stage of the treatment to which I have referred, because it became an important challenge for the analytical work.

In this context, a playful, one could say creative response on my part generates a very significant change in the child's attitude and in the dynamics of the therapeutic process itself, allowing movement in the patient from a repetitive scheme of opposition and confrontation towards a novel, playful and libidinal scenario.

This material is intended to be an invitation to reflect on certain issues concerning the child analyst's technique and interventions during her daily practice with patients with severe disorders when they have already attained a certain level of evolution. It also sets the scene for thinking about the analyst-patient relationship, the transference bond itself being an opportunity for a new encounter with the other.

Brief presentation of the patient and clinical context

Darius is referred to me at the age of 3. He has a diagnosis of a severe childhood disorder which the *DSM-5* classifies under autism spectrum disorders.

After two years of treatment, with sessions taking place twice weekly, favourable evolution occurred. The child had been gradually acquiring the necessary resources for relating with adults and peers. He also used verbal

DOI: 10.4324/9781032614823-7

language appropriately and expressed his experiences in the first person "I" and began to mention a schoolfriend with whom he enjoyed playing. At the age of five he already knew the alphabet and, to my surprise, could read and write. His parents saw positive changes, and this view was shared by his school. However, at this stage of the process, due to his persistent difficulties in organising graphic space and his weak drawing skills, a referral was made for a psychomotor approach. Furthermore, sometimes when he felt very happy he still showed excessive excitement, which was expressed in a degree of tension and lack of control of his limbs. In such situations, he showed mechanical and stereotyped movements, mainly in his arms and hands. Psychic structuring, with the organisation of a mental space and its containing framework for emotional experience, was still in progress.

In his final year of pre-school education, Darius began to show strong oppositional defiance during the sessions, and this attitude extended to his family and school life. He constantly tried to impose his own criteria in an authoritarian and inflexible manner, which caused episodic confusion and chaos. When I did not accede to his demands or his sudden rule changes, he would have loud outbursts of strained shouts and screaming, while deliberately hurling and scattering everything around him. He usually abruptly broke off these scenes when it was time to say goodbye or at other times, which I felt were unpredictable. Adopting an attitude of vigorous provocation, he began trying to transgress boundaries, looking me defiantly in the eye with a clear expectation of confrontation. Sometimes these challenges involved risks, for example trying to touch a table lamp. These situations made us physically grapple with each other, sometimes for much of the session. During this period it was common for him to arrive at the clinic barefoot or without a coat even in the middle of winter, because his parents had been unable to get him to put his shoes or jacket on. Then again, if he was wearing shoes when he arrived, he would repeatedly throw them in the air, risking breaking something. At the end of each session, he usually intentionally left all the material lying around, firmly saying, "I don't want to tidy up," "I'm not going to tidy up." Oppositional defiance, the destructive impulse and authoritarian behaviour arose as expressions of his emergence from the autistic mode.

At the same time, he sporadically began to display quite creative, organised play scenes. Sometimes, he would propose role-plays in which he would be the owner of a restaurant, for example, and I would be the customer he was serving. At other times, he was interested in learning about board games, which he learned quickly but then wanted to impose his own rules.

Darius steadfastly maintained this attitude for many months, which I found overwhelming and very complex as I searched for resources to try and introduce more flexibility into the situation. Despite the anger and discomfort I felt at his attitudes, our goodbyes were usually affectionate, and he sometimes didn't want to leave. On the other hand, when he arrived at the session, and I good-humouredly greeted him and asked him how he was, he would come inside without even looking at me, and his response would be laconic and listless: "Bad". Similarly, when he noticed that he was enjoying an activity, he would abruptly break it off, saying "I don't want to be funny", or with an exaggerated voice and gestures, he would say, "I'm not happy, I'm sad, I am."

Although he was an intelligent child and his resources were expanding, he showed a marked refusal to recognise his capacity to grow, enjoy and learn. "I am zero, zero, zero, zero, zero," he insisted, while at other times he clearly expressed, "I am a boy who doesn't want to grow up . . . no, no, oh no!" His persistent oppositional defiance was also displayed at school and interfered with his learning and performance there. He was about to start his primary education, which was a cause for concern.

I was trying to understand this attitude from different perspectives, and as I found space for it, I was passing it on to him. At first, given the difficulties that Darius presented when he came to the consultation, I wondered whether his oppositional defiance could be an expression of his need for self-reassurance due to a continuing experience of fragility and ego vulnerability. In this sense, the possibility that Darius could say what he wanted and what he did not want could in itself be valued as an evolution and an achievement. From this perspective, I pointed out to him that perhaps saying no made him feel stronger, and that it was very good that he could say what he wanted and what he didn't want. However, I added, there were things that he could not decide because he was a child and the grown-ups get to decide, or because certain things have their own rules for our own safety or so we can play.

Another strand addressed his need for firm and consistent boundaries and a strong and present father figure. At other times, in contrast, I pointed out his oppositional defiance in terms of intrapsychic conflict and in reference to two tendencies he had: firstly, a tendency to grow, which allowed him to learn to read, write and play; and secondly, a tendency, or a part of himself, that did not allow him to grow up because he felt that might mean giving up being his mother's baby, a place he did not seem to want to lose.

However, none of these interventions succeeded in bringing about a change in his attitude or in the dynamics of the sessions. "No, no and no!" Darius always said if I alluded to his oppositional defiance, whether in the analyst-patient dialogue or through the voice of one of the characters in the scenes we play-acted together.

Darius' functioning oscillated considerably. The more resources he acquired, the more vehemently the discourse of "not wanting to grow up" or an image of himself as "a zero-year-old baby" seemed to assert itself. Different elements of the family dynamics overtly and covertly supported this oppositional defiance, which also extended to the functions of his daily life: not wanting to eat, not wanting to go to the toilet, not wanting to sleep, etc. I often interviewed the parents and participated in meetings at his school and with the psychomotor therapist. They asked me for some resources to enable them to work with the child and to soften his intransigent refusal, which prevented him from evolving and learning. As Houzel (2020) argues, this scenario of fluid communication between the parties turned out to be a very important element for the child's evolution and for the continuity of his development and learning process.

From repetition to novelty

In one session during this period, Darius took a large elephant and a smaller one out of a basket of toys and said that they were father and son. "You are the son," he said.

When I asked him what the son was doing, he told me to do whatever I wanted. This put me in a dilemma about which aspects of Darius to incorporate into the scene. Although his most characteristic traits were transgression and confrontation at the time, I chose another path by representing a son-elephant who very energetically and enthusiastically invites his father to play ball. In a post-session reading, it occurred to me that perhaps in doing so I may have been aware of seeing his father as a distant and undemonstrative person, and also the child's expectation of a closer and more pleasurable encounter between them. Darius, responding as if he were the father elephant, accepts the invitation, and we have the two characters play with a little ball together. A desirable and pleasurable father-son bond of playing happily together unfolds in the playful scene. I notice that Darius is enjoying this activity. He is relaxed, laughing and having fun, makes suggestions that enrich the game and does not seem to be as excited as usual when his experiences are very intense. After playing together in this way for a while, I tell him, with a certain degree of complicity:

A: "It looks as if the father and son are having fun playing together."
    He suddenly stops gesturing and loses his animated tone of voice, saying sharply, "They're not having fun."
    I sense from his reply that my comment was ill-timed. My appreciation interfered with the scene in our game and interrupted the child's capacity for enjoyment of a loving and companionable bond between parent and child as it was taking place in the fantasy. Darius immediately picks up the two elephants, wraps them in a piece of wool he finds in his box of materials and in a clear gesture of defiance and provocation looks at me and slides them up the wall, saying that they are making it dirty.
    This sudden change of attitude surprises me. In an attempt to return to the playful dimension, looking at the characters on the wall and then at him, I say, in a calm voice and with a certain tone of intrigue:
    "It looks to me as if they're climbing the mountain. They're tied together with a rope, climbing – just like climbers do."

Darius looks at me, somewhat puzzled by my answer, while stopping the characters with his hands at the top of the wall. I notice that he is unusually interested, so I go on. Looking at the elephants I put on a serious voice, as if I were the father elephant: "Be careful, son, there may be a rockslide there. Be careful, follow me through this passage, it's safer." Suddenly joining in with the story, Darius spontaneously moves the toy animals upwards, as if climbing the wall-mountain. Then, continuing the made-up story and again speaking as if I were the father, I tell the son to go ahead on a path so that I can see him in case he needs help. Following the story, Darius then changes the position of the elephants on the wall, placing the elephant-son in front of the father.

Then, plainly invested in this story, he asks me what else is on the mountain.

Trying to imagine the scenario and attempting to offer a range of possibilities, I tell him that there might be eagles' nests high up in the rocks, or there might be a lizard in a cave by the road, or there might be snow on the top of the mountain making it impassable, and there might even be a volcano on the other side, so no one can go there, either.

Darius listens to me attentively and then stops moving the animals any higher up. He looks at me, and pointing at a spot even higher up on the wall, he asks, "So they can't go there?"

A: "And no," I answer. "If in our game there is snow or a volcano there, then they can't go there."

Darius then makes the animals avoid that path. He then asks me, "What will happen next?"

A: "I don't know," I say, deep in thought. "What could it be?"

"You tell me," he replies. I add that they may have walked a long way and may need to rest, and that the father must have been carrying something to drink in his backpack for the two of them, as climbers do.

Darius seems to agree. He rests the elephants on the table, saying that the father brought chocolate for the son and that he is going to drink coffee. He acts out this situation. We then invent a dialogue between the father and son elephants, who talk about how far they have walked, and the things they have seen along the way. Finally, intending to finish the story and seeing that it is time to say our goodbyes, I put on the father's voice and have him show his son that there are some clouds gathering, and that we have to get down the mountain quickly.

Darius proposes a twist to the story, looking at me very seriously, saying that they are caught in the rain on the road.

A: "Well," I say, trying to readjust to the new situation, "then they might be in danger of slipping. They'll have to go to a shelter to wait out the rain. And where might that be? Where could the shelter be?" I ask.

P: "I know!" he says enthusiastically, going to fetch some blocks and building something on the table. He then moves the elephants there.

Then, again in father elephant's voice, I say, "Look, son, there is the shelter", looking at Darius expectantly. He looks at me and nods, as if to get me to go on with the scene. I find his answers very stimulating. I then continue as the father elephant:

"I think there's some smoke coming out of the chimney, perhaps my climbing friends are there." I look at Darius and in my own tone of voice I ask him, "Do you think so?" He nods again. I see that he is interested, engaged in the game and expectant. He then places the elephants inside the "shelter" he built with the blocks. There I play the role of the father elephant again, introducing my elephant son to my friends, and proudly recounting the adventures we have had together in the mountains.

Darius tells me that the son wants to climb higher. However, seeing that it is time to say goodbye, again speaking in the father's voice, I tell my son and climbing friends that a storm is forecast on the radio and that everyone has to leave the hut quickly and go the rest of the way down the mountain. "Come on, let's go!" I say in the role of the father.

Darius brings the elephants down from the table, while we imagine that the climbing friends are also coming down. On his own initiative, he then has them say goodbye. "The elephants are going to the car to get home," he says, "and the little elephant is going to tell his mother about his adventure in the mountains."

I see that Darius is very happy and calm. When I start collecting up the play equipment to put in its box, as I had been doing each session for the past few months, he very willingly says, "No, I'll put it away", as if this were completely normal.

After we say goodbye, I hear him enthusiastically telling his father that we played at elephants climbing the mountain.

Playful and emotional display

In the following sessions, Darius proposes carrying on with this game, and together we add new details, for example a map of the mountain, where we place a cave, a waterfall, and so on. "I'm going to play with the elephants," he would say. "This is for the map," he added, as he carefully tore out a sheet of paper from his pad. "This is for the shelter," he said, reaching for some blocks, "and this is for the waterfall," he remarked, placing a cushion against an armchair to form a slope. He suggested, "You make the map of the cave and the waterfall, okay?"

A: "Well, what are you going to do?"
P: "I'm going to put the safety harness on the elephants for climbing," he said, referring to the wool that had bound the two elephants together since the game had first started. "And the elephants need a car. I'm going to make a car." He does so using blocks, as he keeps on telling me what he is doing. "As the son is big, let's put him like this," he adds,

mentioning the seat for the son, the car windows and a seat for the father. When he has finished, he very happily shows me what he has built and points to where the engine and fuel are.

For months, with intervals of sporadic scenes of oppositional defiance, loud screaming and play crying, Darius continued to develop this game of the elephant father and his son, adding multiple variants and new characters. Thus, for example, he added a lion who was a friend of the father elephant and a tiger who was "little elephant's" friend. Over the course of several sessions, he creates a sequence in which the parents build the children a tree house on the mountain near the shelter. Darius asks me to be the parents who stay in the refuge, while the children – who he works with his hands – enjoy being grown up and being able to explore the mountain on their own. In these "explorations" Darius invents various situations that the children face on their way, in the form of obstacles or challenges to be overcome. For example, they discover a lake and go swimming in it, a cave inhabited by bats, etc. In subsequent sessions, there are sequences in which the children are grown up and living alone in another country. When this occurs, he asks me to help him build the children's two-storey house with blocks. He then furnishes the building with beds, a dining table etc. Then he also builds a plane that the children fly to visit their parents in the mountains, which in other versions of the game will be a mobile home. In these scenes, the parents, whom Darius asks me to work, hear the sound of the engine and happily come out of the shelter to greet their children, whom they see as grown up and capable of doing many things.

After the summer holidays, when the school year was about to start, Darius returned to the stories about the elephants. Secondary characters continued to be developed, and the story took many twists and turns.

In one session which took place in his first few weeks of starting primary school, he arrived in a good mood, greeted me warmly and went straight to the blackboard. He wrote his name and those of some of his friends, asking me for some of the letters when he was unsure. He notices that there are other names that end with the letter "o", like his (Darío, in original Spanish language), and that catches his attention. I tell him that's right, several boys' names end with an "o", and we write some of them together. He then tells me the names of other friends, distinguishing them from those ending with the letter "o". Although his handwriting is uneven in size and the space is not sufficiently organised, I am surprised at how well he can write, and I tell him this. I also add that he is showing me that he has a lot of friends and that must make him feel very happy. He tells me that there are also others who are not his friends because they hit people, and tells me about his friends at the summer club and other children there who were prone to hitting. I tell him that it is important to know who his friends are and who are not his friends.

Darius says nothing and reflects. When I ask him what he is thinking about, he smiles rather shyly and mischievously, saying, "I'm thinking about Romi. She's beautiful!" He tells me that she is a girl in his class and that she is a very good friend of his. "I'm going to write her a letter," he says. He finds a sheet of paper and begins writing, saying the words aloud: *"Good morning Romi, Fede, Juani and Joaco, I love you, because I like to play and eat with you and go to your house. And I like it when you come to my house. I'm writing a letter because I am missing you and I like the fact that you are very big when you are in primary school. I love you."*

At the end of the session I notice he is moved. I, too, am pleasantly touched by his evolution, his ability to enjoy his friends and his demonstrations of affection.

Darius folds his letter up and takes it with him and shows it to his father when he comes to collect him.

The transferential link: an opportunity for a new encounter with the other

The material presented is intended to be an invitation to reflect on certain aspects of the child analyst's technique, form of intervention and the transferential bond itself as an opportunity for a new encounter with the other in children who present a serious disorder in early childhood.

I have deliberately omitted to mention details of the patient's history and the early stages of the process in order to focus more on the clinical situation. However, as the present case concerns a young child with a serious disorder, it is to be assumed that difficulties in early bonds hindered communication, intersubjective experience and, therefore, the subjectivation process, beyond the aetiology of these situations, which is always complex and is multiply determined (Alvarez, 2020).

Furthermore, it is worth noting that during the stage of the analytical process to which I am referring, there are significant developments in Darius' oppositional defiance, authoritarian attitude and confrontation seeking, which in themselves imply recognition of the other. At the same time, these behaviours are also an expression of the child's trust in the analytic bond and in his analyst's ability to contain his destructive impulses, to guard against them and to her enduring vitality (Winnicott, 1971a). Moreover, his affectionate farewells in each session demonstrate an analytical bond with libidinal characteristics.

In this context, Darius' initiative to play with the two elephants, telling me to be the son and asking me to do as I wish, is an invitation on his part for me to become emotionally involved in the scene. That is to say, an invitation to engage my capacity to perceive the affects involved in the parent-child relationship which he is presenting.

After the ball game between the characters and my ill-timed intervention in pointing out what fun the elephants were having, Darius reacts provocatively, placing the toy elephants on the wall and defiantly warning me that they are "making a mess" of it. My response at that time in developing the scene of the father and son climbing the mountain promotes a very significant change in the child. Darius abandons the concrete setting of his destructive impulse – to make the wall dirty – and accepts my invitation to return to the dimension of play. That is, to the realm of representation, imagination and fantasy (Winnicott, 1967, 1971b).

Within the game scene a significant creative and emotional process thus unfolds on different levels. Firstly, he adds content that enriches the story and the relationship between the two characters. His proposals show the evolution and growth of the elephant-child that is standing in for him and a close and affectionate bond with an elephant-father, who encourages and celebrates his son's autonomy and growth.

Secondly, in his developing game, Darius is trying out quite complex ego functions. For example, he uses a map, an element that delimits, orients and allows representation and recognition of a space. He also plans activities at the beginning of each session, sorts and organises the material to be used for different functions, and divides tasks between us both. All these capacities – distinguishing, classifying, planning and organising – are evidence of greater ego resources and psychic structuring. In this sense, his reference to a house made by parents for their children could be seen to represent a delimited psychic space of his own.

Throughout successive sessions, the two of them – analyst and patient – create a story about a relationship between two protagonists from two generations. It is an asymmetrical relationship, just as the analytic relationship itself is, and it is a hopeful story, of a parent (mother-analyst) who is capable of caring for the child and who also shows confidence in his capacity to evolve and forge his own path, opening up towards new libidinal objects.

At the same time, in his social life Darius is expanding the world of his personal relationships and his emotional experience of bonds. The emotive letter he writes to his friends shows his capacity and willingness to engage in activities with them, play together and visit each other's homes, as well as expressing his affection for them. His social life is enriched by new signs of change and evolution. The transferential bond takes on an affectionate and collaborative quality during these processes.

Finally, I would like to discuss a particular aspect of the play scene about the father and son climbing the mountain from which the story develops. The fact that I myself spontaneously proposed this scene, rather than the patient, is a detail which I consider merits reflection. A number of questions come to mind. Did this scene of mine intrude into the child's play? Did presenting it force a point that the patient was not expressing? Or on the contrary, could it be said to have represented latent content that may have been present within the child but which for various reasons had not found a form of expression?

Darius' response, appropriating and engaging in the story, enriching it with new details, and his subsequent evolution, make me inclined to believe the latter possibility. In other words, I believe that for Darius, the suggested play scene acquired a certain interpretative value, representing the patient's own expectation of being able to leave behind a representation of himself as a "zero-year-old" child (in other words of emerging from the remnants of the autistic world), to open up to new paths, to broaden his range of experiences, and to face the adventure and the challenge of growing up (climbing the mountain).

My understanding of this spontaneously acted out scene of mine is that it arose out of the analytic encounter: the analyst's emotional readiness to perceive the patient's needs and to intervene accordingly is considered an inherent element of the analytic encounter. It is therefore an intervention in which the analyst's imagination and creativity come into play in order to find ways of communicating with deep aspects of the child's suffering that have not yet been described in words.

This perspective implies allowing a condition of dynamism and adaptability to enter into the setting of approaches for young children with severe pathologies, in order to be able to offer the patient tools that allow him to continue in his growth and evolutionary processes. As Urtubey (1999) states, the psychoanalytical setting is not only defined by its physical or temporal/frequential characteristics, but also by the asymmetrical roles of the two participants and, by extension, by the analyst's internal setting in her readiness to listen to the patient, which, when working with children, is extended to play and other expressions of their experiences.

In this regard, also of interest is Quinodoz's (1992) concept of the setting as an entity through which the analyst's containing function is expressed. This author sees the setting as an instrument with effects for the patient which lie rather more in the active character of the container than in the rules that comprise it.

To conclude these reflections, we could say that with regard to analytic work with young children with severe disorders, paradoxically the possibility of flexibility and adaptability of the setting allows the analytic process to develop, transference and countertransference being fundamental elements of it. Thus, as a result of the emotional contact and creativity that arises between both the analyst and patient in the analytic encounter, the transferential bond becomes a transformative opportunity for the child in the experiences with the other.

References

Alvarez, A. (2020, November). A propósito del elemento de déficit en niños con autismo: psicoterapia basada en el psicoanálisis y factores del desarrollo [On the element of deficit in children with autism: Psychotherapy based on psychoanalysis and developmental factors]. *eipea Magazine*, (9), 8–18.

De Urtubey, L. (1999). *El encuadre y sus elementos [The framework and its elements].* https://www.apuruguay.org/apurevista/1990/1688724719998904.pdf.

Houzel, D. (2020). Aportaciones del psicoanálisis al tratamiento de los niños autistas [Contributions of psychoanalysis to the treatment of autistic children]. *eipea Magazine*, (8), 8–14.

Quinodoz, D. (1992). The psychoanalytic setting as the instrument of the container function. *International Journal of Psychoanalysis, 73,* 627–635.

Winnicott, D. (1967). Chapter 3: Playing, a theoretical statement. In *Playing and reality*. London: Tavistock Publications, pp. 38–52.

Winnicott, D. W. (1971a). The use of an object and relating through identifications. *Playing and Reality, 17,* 86–94. London. Tavistock Publications.

Winnicott, D. W. (1971b). Playing: Creative activity and the search for the self. *Playing and Reality, 17,* 53–64. London: Tavistock Publications.

6 The analyst and the parents of the young child with autism spectrum disorder

The physical presence of parents forms a specific and inevitable part of child psychoanalysis. The space that the analyst does or does not allocate the parents throughout the process is determined on the basis of a concept of the early psyche and the construction of subjectivity and the corresponding technique. The different perspectives in this field are therefore in line with the broad theoretical outlines of our discipline.

In the case of Melanie Klein, for example, child analysis focuses exclusively on the patient and his or her inner world, and the analyst's encounters with the parents are seen as an invasion of the child's analytic space (Klein, 1932). In this context, parental involvement is limited to the start of treatment and only serves the purpose of gathering information. It is not considered essential, although it is also not actively discouraged (Bleichmar and Sigal de Rosenberg, 1995). Meltzer (1967) also reaffirms the position of focusing analytic work on the child, suggesting that the analyst remain as politely distant from the parents as possible, complying exclusively with the minimum social norms to be expected.

In contrast, Winnicott (1945) introduces the idea that the external world, as represented by the mother figure, forms an essential part of the structure of the early psyche, and argues that both the child and its parents play a part in the young child's incipient psyche (Winnicott, 1945, 1960). In this way, what the author calls "early basic environmental provision" will come to occupy a central place in his theory as a necessary element to enable the processes of emotional development and ego-integration in the child (1962). Winnicott further extends this environmental influence to the prospect of success of the child's treatment, considering that the child's mental health cannot be established without good enough parental or maternal care (1962).

On the other hand, Mannoni (1976) and Dolto (1973), from a Lacanian perspective, also attribute a relevant place to the parents in the child's analytical process by emphasising the importance of their unconscious desire in the child's symptom.

These different historical perspectives are equally applicable to the approach taken for the patients in question. At present, there are numerous

DOI: 10.4324/9781032614823-8

diverging strands of thought on whether and how to integrate parents into the analytical process of the young child with autistic disorder, with no consensus.

Contemporary authors, such as Bush de Ahumada and Ahumada (2015), influenced by Klein, Meltzer and Tustin, do not see the need to involve parents in the child's treatment (p. 67). Instead, they receive them only occasionally and under certain circumstances: during the initial assessment, once or twice a year throughout the process if the parents require it or if difficulties present and, finally, parents are invited to end-of-treatment interviews (p. 67). These authors use this technique in all child analyses, without modifying it in function of the severity of the patient's pathology or the age of the child (p. 67).

In contrast to this position, Joyce (2010) holds that the analyst's work with the parents is an indispensable condition for the analytical process of children with autistic disorder. Alvarez (2020) also stresses the importance of working with parents, and goes so far as to propose the possibility of working with the child within the context of the family (p. 15). Cecchi, extending the range of possibilities further (2013, 2021), suggests the need for family therapy at the same time as child analysis.

In my experience, given the child's physical and emotional dependence on his or her parents, I have come to see them as decisive not only to enable the continuity and regularity of the treatment but also to generate certain conditions in the family dynamic itself that enable active support of the patient's gradual evolution. Moreover, beyond any difficulties or resistances that may arise for the parents, integrating them in the child's analytical process tends to favour a complex transferential scenario, which benefits the work with the patient and the bond between the child and his or her parents.

In this context, the presence and participation of the mother or father in clinical sessions with the child contribute to shaping a setting and a technique that are adapted to the patient's age and pathology, especially at the start of the process or at certain times when the situation and/or the child requires it. In the same vein, periodic interviews with parents at regular intervals of varying frequency form part of a flexible strategy aimed at promoting greater understanding and affective proximity to the child's experiences and needs. Thus, when treatment of the young child with a severe disorder is going well, this impacts the parents, who become actively involved in the process of change and evolution.

Parents in clinical sessions with the child at the start of the analytical process

It is in itself clinically significant whether a young child enters the first consultations with the analyst alone or accompanied by a parent, and likewise when the child has a severe disorder. Given the young age of the patients in question, it is only to be expected that they will need to be accompanied by a parent for the first interviews, or the parents themselves want to accompany their young child to an unfamiliar place and a person outside their family environment. Conversely, on the occasions when the parents are not present in the room with the child during the first interview, as was the case with the girl I called Matilde (Chapter 1), I considered that the physical distance between her and her mother could indicate an affective distance.

Far from seeing the presence of the mother or father in the initial consultations with the child as a problem, or something that could stand in the way of the analyst-patient encounter, I see their presence as an opportunity which allows the analyst to observe the dynamics of a mother-child or father-child bond and their effects on the early psyche. I shall attempt to illustrate these aspects with the following vignette. On the other hand, it should be added that this setting in itself also shapes an intervention scenario with its own characteristics.

Teo, aged 2 years and a few months, arrives for his first consultation with his mother. He has a diagnosis of autistic spectrum disorder. His gaze is vague and does not fix on anything. He does not seek or respond to my gaze. Nor does he look at his mother. He does not utter any sounds or words. As he enters the consulting room, he begins to aimlessly and rapidly run from one side to the other. When he manages to stop, he stands in front of the material on a low table and impulsively throws it hard against the wall. He immediately goes back to running around. The mother, sitting on the floor, talks to him, telling him that there are some toy cars the same as the ones he likes. In an attempt to invite him to play, she moves the toy cars towards him in different directions, following him around the room. Teo ignores them, continuing to rapidly and unpredictably run back and forth. I ask the mother a question in a deliberately soft and slow tone of voice, and she looks at me to answer, taking her eyes off the child. I notice that Teo sneaks up on one of the toy cars with the intention of pushing it across the floor. Attentive to this situation, I continue talking to the mother and looking at her, and I also turn my gaze towards the child, observing his initiative. The mother follows my gaze. When she sees Teo approaching the toy car, she suddenly bursts into loud, forced laughter, perhaps because she is pleased and is trying to encourage him to play, and abruptly emits loud, high-pitched cries of "*Yeaaaaaahhh!!! Cooeeee! Yeeaaahhh!!!!*" At the same time, with a sudden show of physicality, she puts a lot of toy cars in front of the child. Everything that has happened in these brief moments surprises and disturbs me. Teo immediately drops the toy car in his hand and hurries away, wandering around the consulting room, again aimlessly.

As Álvarez (2020) puts it, "knowledge about the nature of early mother-infant dialogue can help clinicians to understand and treat the communication difficulties of the autistic child" (p. 15). In this scene between

Teo and his mother, which may well be a paradigmatic scene of the way this dyad functions, there is no possibility of synchrony being experienced (Brazelton et al., 1974) or of affective attunement (Tronick, 2007), which the young child – the infant – needs in order to recognise its own emotional states with the other and in the other (Stern, 1985; Gergely and Watson, 1996). On the contrary, there is predominantly misunderstanding and disconnection between the two protagonists, despite the mother's willingness and attempt to relate to her son, making use of the resources she possesses. Excess in the mother inhibits the child's incipient initiative, *the spontaneous gesture*, in Winnicott's words (1960). For multiple possible reasons, which involve unconscious aspects and are beyond her control, the maternal response fails to take on a structuring function for Teo which would allow him to generate resources to contain his arousal and process experiences. Instead, the child is left alone and seized by the strength of his impulses, while his mother, unaware of the effect of her reaction, feels bewildered, helpless and frustrated.

According to Bleichmar (1984, p. 105), in child analysis the child's own disturbance must be worked on and, at the same time, the conditions that generate it. This position takes on particular importance in relation to the patients in question. The process of psychic structuring of the child does not take place in mythical times but in real times (Bleichmar, p. 108). The baby's encounter with its mother, its parents and other significant adults generates structuring movements in the construction of subjectivity. Conversely, if the conditions of a bond that disrupts the young child's incipient psyche are not discontinued or changed, then they will continue to have a negative impact on the child's functioning, with the risk of further disorganisation and the accentuation of extreme defensive mechanisms of isolation or disconnection.

Considering the communication deficit presented by the patients to whom I am referring, Álvarez (2020) suggests that

> whatever the combination of factors that has left the child on the road to autism, the conditions for recovery may lie in encouraging a capacity for interaction in the patient, taking into account his or her level of development, which is possibly at a very early stage.
>
> (p. 4)

In this sense, the analyst's initiative and actions in seeking contact through verbal and non-verbal aspects, as well as her sensitive responses to the child's limited gestural expressions, form part of a strategy aimed at generating and fostering interaction and the analyst-patient bond (Chapter 2).

Moreover, when these exchanges between the analyst and the child take place in the presence of the mother or father, then a new element is added to the dynamics of the session, which generates new repercussions.

A multiple transference scenario

Once help has been requested for the child, demands coming from both sides, that is, from the child and also from his or her parents, converge and interrelate. This initial activity, which is characteristic of child psychoanalysis, gives rise to a complex scenario of multiple and reciprocal transference which involves and produces effects on all participants (Mannoni, 1976). As proposed by Armesto et al. (2017), this multiple or extended transference field, which includes the parents' transference to the analyst, unfolds in a privileged way in interventions with young children in the presence of their parents. This aspect has existed since analytic work with children began. Thus, for example, in Freud's encounter with Little Hans with his father present (Freud, 1909), the aspects of the father's transference lead him to feel addressed by Freud's intervention, even though it was aimed not at him but at the child. In other words, through his own transference to Freud, the child's manifestations acquire a new meaning for the father (Armesto et al., 2017).

Effects of this transferential dynamic of the parents towards the analyst have also been observed in previous chapters as, for example, in the clinical sessions with the 15-month-old baby I have called Juanita and her mother (Chapter 3), or in the initial stages of Fabian's analytical process, which took place in his father's presence (Chapter 4). In fact, on that occasion, at a certain moment the father spontaneously took up the analyst's initiative of drawing on the blackboard, and he himself drew an image of the pirate ship. This had a favourable effect on the child and also gave the analyst an insight into his interests, thus favouring the analyst-patient encounter and the evolution of the therapy itself. In both situations, even though the analyst is pointing things out to the child, the parent present in the session also has their attention drawn to them and acts accordingly, on the basis of a new portrayal of the child's limited forms of expression, which allows the possibility of a new bond beginning to form. Similarly, Álvarez (2020), in her work with a little girl with an autistic disorder who is accompanied by her mother, emphasised the child's desire to share her pleasure with her mother. This made the mother happy and physically willing to engage in an affectionate hug with the child, which then actually occurred before the analyst's eyes (p. 15).

From this perspective, increased affective proximity of the parent to the child's experiences and needs, and along with this, the possibility of generating a new encounter, does not come from taking a pedagogical approach with them, nor from intervening with instructions on how to specifically encourage the field of interaction. Instead, this movement on the part of the parents is an effect of the dynamics of a transference which involves them. By definition, every psychoanalytic intervention includes transference, and along with this a complex scenario of identifications. While the analyst does not interpret the parents' transference to herself (Zusman de Arbiser,

2009, p. 475), the presence of the mother or father in the session along with the child – with their transference to the analyst as a backdrop – causes the parents to enter into processes of identification with the analyst's sensitivity and the possibility of communication with the child during the session.

This position is a departure from the approach of Bush de Ahumada and Ahumada (2015, p. 67) in considering that the achievements acquired by the child in the analytical setting are transferred directly to the family environment. It also distances itself from these authors with respect to the idea that the analyst's own work with the parents could interfere with the "quality of care" given to the patient (2015, p. 67). On the other hand, the technical modality that I intend to illustrate is closer to Álvarez (2020) suggestion regarding the importance of working with the parents of the child with an autistic disorder. This author recounts clinical situations with young children in the presence of the mother and points out the need to sensitise parents to respond to weak or immature signals from the child that are not clearly expressed in order to avoid further estrangement between the child and parents (p. 14). In my experience, the presence of parents in the initial sessions with the child generates an intervention scenario that promotes subjectivity for both the child and the parents.

In this context, one aspect that deserves reflection is the length of time that would be considered necessary or opportune to maintain a setting that integrates the presence of the mother or father accompanying the child in the clinical sessions at the start of the treatment. Or in other words, what conditions would lead to an analytic space for the young child with a severe disorder, alone with the analyst? As in so many other aspects of psychoanalysis, I realise that a single, generalisable answer is not possible. On the contrary, the conditions of this change need to be analysed in each particular situation, in the course of a process that involves both the patient and his or her parents, and perhaps also the analyst. However, I have noticed that the child's subtle expressions of expectation of meeting the analyst and the equipment, as well as the initiative to take toys home from the consulting room or to stop asking the parent present in the session to intervene, were manifestations of a certain recognition of the analytic space as his or her own. As for the parents, the introduction of resources in communication with the child and the perception and appreciation of details of the patient's gestures, which implied a certain flexibility in contact with the other and, above all, with the analyst, was making them increasingly confident in the analytical framework and in the person of the analyst. However, from my clinical perception, I often noticed that the child's movement towards appropriation of the analytic space was often expressed earlier in the patient than in the parents. On the other hand, they tended to show some resistance to my proposal to work alone with the child, which took on a certain connotation of loss. Sometimes parents even commented, very emotionally, that these clinical sessions were the first spaces in which they had been able to share and enjoy an encounter with their child. For my part, while recognising the legitimacy of these approaches, I sensed that perhaps the parents' greater sensitivity to the child's difficulties and experiences of vulnerability could awaken more primary transferential aspects in them which could be traced back to their own childhood experiences of vulnerability and helplessness.

As in all transferential phenomena, the infantile is at play in the transference from the parents to the analyst. In these sessions with the young child in the presence of the parent, I have often found myself a spectator to brief affectionate exchanges or simple playful activities which the child and the parent shared and enjoyed together in front of me. As Álvarez (2020) points out in relation to the little girl and her mother who give each other an affectionate hug, sparking joy in everyone present in the session, including the analyst (p. 15), these encounters that were pleasurable for the child and her parent also generated the same sensation in me, which we then shared.

Based on my experience, given the transferential mobilisation that can be generated in parents by their presence in the clinical sessions of a young child with an autistic disorder, I ask myself: does the parent present in the session need to be seen by a third party – an analyst who is transferentially valued, who enables and recognises them in their parental role, and in their capacity to generate a new encounter with their child? Could we then consider this transferential scenario as a potential opportunity for change, with a certain restorative effect on the bond between the child and the parent present in the session?

Parents and the process of change

In my clinical experience, the presence and participation of the parents in the analytical process of the young child with severe pathology has been a determining element in facilitating the patient's evolution. I agree with Bleichmar's (1984) view on the analysis of children in general that, in the approach to the children with whom we are dealing, it is essential to open a space for the parents that is their own, in which the positioning modes and identification offerings towards the child are re-signified, in order to thus create conditions which enable consolidation and promote the process of subjectivation that begins in the analytical setting (p. 106).

In this sense, the technical resource of regular interviews with the parents is a prompt to listen and exchange ideas, which is an opportunity to mitigate any insecurities, anxieties and conflicts that the parents may experience in the face of the child's gradual evolution. These spaces also allow the analyst to transmit experiences and functions that the patient manifests during the sessions, and which the parents are unable to perceive, or cannot understand. In general, despite the parents' limitations and resistance, such communications allow for a certain flexibility in the representation they have of the child and its disorder, which allows the patient mobility in relation to the space it and its pathology occupy in the family. Sometimes, the mobilisation which occurs in the mother or father as a result of these encounters, as well as the experience of analytical listening and the appreciation of the child's treatment, can lead the parents to seek out a therapeutic space of their own with another professional outside the child's analytical setting.

Thus, when the child's analytic process is successful, it has transformative effects not only on the patient, but also on his or her parents and on the family dynamic itself. Conversely, when certain aspects rooted in the parents' infantile sexuality prevail and invade the child's analytical space, then obstacles arise, which have a negative impact on the patient and his or her evolutionary process. I will attempt to illustrate these aspects by returning to Teo's story, which I started in this chapter:

> After two years of an analytical process of three weekly sessions, **Teo, aged 4**, showed favourable evolution. At that point, he had been attending the sessions alone for over a year. He no longer showed episodes of disconnection and isolation and, although his resources were still limited, he showed some initiative in contact with others. He had incorporated words and verbal expressions, which he used with communicative intent and with a sharable meaning, and he referred to himself in the first person "I". He generally came to the sessions in a very good mood and was affectionate. His interests were still quite elementary for his age, but he enjoyed sharing certain playful activities together, which although they tended to be repetitive were gradually expanding with new proposals, made either by him or by me. At school, he recognised the names of some of the children in his class, whom he identified as "my friends". Sometimes, he would ask me to draw them on the blackboard, while he would identify each of these figures by name. His perception and mastery of his own body and enjoyment of his movements were also gradually increasing. Certain board games with puzzles or animal figures were also incorporated into the session. There involved the capacity for sequencing, organisation or turn taking, which Teo remembered and respected. These were all signs of a growing ego organisation.

However, I noted with concern that as the child gradually evolved, his parents were becoming markedly more distant towards the analytical process. They were beginning to show difficulties in bringing Teo to his sessions as well as in attending interviews that I had invited them to, which eventually had to be cancelled or postponed. This parents' distance also manifested in relation to the child's experiences. In the meetings we did manage to have, they highlighted his evolution, but at the same time their conversation remained at a superficial level, and they did not really get involved in Teo's problems or accept the true dimension of his emotional needs, which they were thus unable to respond to.

One Monday, when I opened the door to welcome him, unusually I saw that his mother had brought him. After greeting each other at the door, she says to me, in front of the child: "I came because I wanted to tell you that we split up. Teo already knows, we have already told him. It happened at the weekend. Teo's father moved to his mother's house, and the boy spent the night with him yesterday. It went well."

I am absolutely astonished. I look at Teo, who is standing still next to his mother, silent, and gazing at me fixedly. Perhaps he senses my surprise. "His aunt is coming to pick him up," adds his mother, with a friendly smile, and leaves. Teo runs into the consulting room. I follow him, as I try to recover from the shock of the news of his parents' separation and, along with this, the trivial way his mother told me about such an important change in the child's life.

Instead of saying something and suggesting what we should play, as Teo usually did, he lies face-down on the couch and pulls a large cushion over himself, covering almost his entire body. It makes me very sad.

A: "What a difficult situation this is that your mum told me about, Teo. There are so many important changes for you at home," I say, coming closer and sitting down next to him.

The child stands up, runs quickly to his play equipment box lying on a low table, and deliberately throws and scatters its entire contents with great force. He shrieks loudly, then settles into an armchair, in a foetal position. None of this had happened in previous sessions. I understand this to be a form of expressing his reaction to the new situation.

A: "You are very angry about what is happening. Maybe it all makes you feel insecure."

He asks me to drape a small blanket lying at the foot of the couch over the arms of the armchair where he is curled up, which then forms a kind of roof over him. From that point on he will refer to this space as "the little house". He puts his thumb in his mouth and sucks it, staring blankly into nothingness. He is conveying his anguish, loneliness and helplessness.

After a few moments, I address him, in a soft, slow voice.

A: "It seems to me that you are feeling lonely and scared. Maybe you wonder how things will be now with Mum and Dad."
T: "I don't know!" he shouts in reply. He immediately stands up and begins to gather some game figures that were scattered on the floor. "There's one missing!" he shouts, as he reaches for one of the figures under the armchair.
A: "Yes, Teo, there's one missing," I say to him. "Because Mum and Dad told you that they won't both be at home together anymore, and you understood very well that one of them will be missing."

He once more forcefully throws and scatters the game figurines. His face tightens in a twisted grimace. I notice the mechanical and stereotyped movements of his hands, like he used to make at the start of treatment, more than two years ago. I am shocked and saddened. I see that he is suffering and trying to process the situation with his fragile resources.

He unexpectedly lets out a very loud scream, which then turns into a prolonged and painful wailing. At the same time, he starts banging his head back and forth between the armchair and the wall. I go over to him and hold his head. I tell him that he is feeling very sad and very angry and that he is showing me that all these things that are happening hurt him and wound him, but that we are going to take care that he doesn't hit himself in this way.

"I want to do it!" he shouts very loudly, trying again to hit his head, with jerky movements. I stop him, holding him tightly.

Teo quickly stands up and, with a fake and exaggerated smile, runs back and forth at breakneck, dizzying speed, just like he used to in the first consultations. He is staring into space, and his face remains scrunched into grotesque expressions. He suddenly throws himself hard on the divan, curls up and covers himself with the cushion that covers his body. He absently sucks his thumb. He seems very distressed. Sometimes he briefly glances in my direction, then covers his head and face again. I think about what to say to him to try to comfort him in some way, but I can't think of anything. I myself am also still under the impact of the new situation, which is totally unexpected.

After a few minutes, he gets up from the couch and wanders around. "But I want to go home," he says, very sadly, perhaps thinking of the house he used to share with both his parents.

A: "And yes, to your house where Mum and Dad were. How hard it is for you to go through so many changes, Teo."

Teo: "Yes, how hard for me."

A: "You feel you have lost your home with Mum and Dad, and you are sad."

Teo: "Very," he says and goes to the armchair, where he again adopts the foetal position, and asks me to cover him with the blanket to make "the little house".

Despite my trying to get in touch with Teo's parents, weeks pass without them responding to my calls for an interview, either together or separately. When at last I did manage to, the outlook was not very encouraging. There was a prevalence of infantile aspects in them, making them inflexible and unresponsive. The new scenario of family dynamics was chaotic, and Teo's parents could not understand the significant disruptive effect this had on their child's fragile psychic functioning. Teo expressed his discomfort in the sessions, and he tried to process the new experiences with his fragile resources. At the same time, and also as a consequence of the change in the family context, he began to often skip sessions because there was no one to bring him or due to a lack of coordination between his parents. The child went back and forth from one house to the other with unrealistic and changing schedules, which disrupted his routines, activities and rest.

In a session that takes place two months after the couple's separation, Teo asks me to help him complete a puzzle which we used to play with. Between the two of us, we put the pieces together on the couch, as we had done so many times before. This time, however, he assembles one half, which he places on the left, and leaves a space separating these figures from the other half, which is then assembled on the right. The two parts of the puzzle are separated by a space between them.

"This is missing," he says, pointing to the empty space in the middle.

A: "The two parts are separated, just like Mum and Dad."
Teo: "This is missing!!!! Missingl!!!" he loudly adds, bursting into an anguished cry.
A: "Yes, Teo, Mummy is missing when you're with Daddy, and Daddy is missing when you're with Mummy. And that's very hard for you," I tell him, in a slow and calm voice.
Teo: "Noooo!!!!!!" he shouts, with an angry expression on his face, as he quickly and forcefully moves an armchair from one side of the consulting room to the other.
A: "Maybe right now, like the armchair, you feel yourself going from one place to another, from the house with Mum, to Grandma's house, where Dad now lives. This all makes you very angry."

The child climbs onto the other armchair, which is still in place, and asks me to cover him with "the blanket". He says it is "the little house". After a few moments, he stands up and goes over to the couch containing the puzzle which has been divided into two halves. He tries to put the two parts together, but the pieces fall off and scatter. He picks up some of these pieces from the floor and throws them down again, this time deliberately and with great force.

He himself then drops from the couch to the floor, as if inert. His facial expression is tense, his mouth is skewed to one side in an exaggerated grimace, he is staring into space and his hands are showing marked stereotypical movements. It is a very distressing sight. I see that he is suffering a great deal.

T: "It can't be, it can't be," he says sadly, lying on the floor. He then stops and tries to put the puzzle back together again, the pieces of which fall off again. He looks at me and asks, "How can we do it?"
A: "You're asking for my help to put together, to build something that will allow you to continue growing, as you've been doing, Teo," I tell him while we are inserting puzzle pieces together.

He suddenly opens his mouth, emitting anguished moans. Again, he throws the pieces with force, and they scatter on the floor once more. He says, "There are two missing."

A: "There are two missing: what is missing is for Mum and Dad to agree to help you feel more secure and enable you to grow up?"

Teo sticks out his tongue with a tense expression and moves around the consulting room throwing everything in his path. He continues to emit pitiful sounds, like moans that fade away: "Aaaaaaaaaaaaaahhhh". Then he lies down on the couch, picks up two blocks of wood that he finds randomly on the floor and bangs them together with great force and gestures of tension. He slips and falls, as do all the blocks on the couch.
   "I fell," he says, plaintively whimpering.

A: "You are showing me that everything that is happening with Mum and Dad makes you experience very, very strong feelings that make you fall into disorganisation and sadness. We are going to try to help you feel better."

He quickly climbs under the couch.

A: "Another little house, so you feel protected from all the strong feelings you are having."
T: "I behaved myself, I'm going to go to school, I go to Grandma's house, Dad's not there. Dad's not there because he works a lot, I go home with Mum." He suddenly starts intoning monotonously, mechanically and very fast, perhaps in an attempt to organise himself, "Aaaah, aargh, one is missing," adding in a pitiful voice and immensely sad voice, "aaaaaaaaah, aaaargh."
A: "Aaaaaah, aaargh, so many things that hurt so much and that you are trying to understand. Why is Dad no longer at home? Why do they take you back and forth?"
T: "I'm very sad," he says with a lot of feeling and looking at me from under the couch. "Dad is never around."

The emotional climate of the session is very distressing. Teo has lost much of his ability to contain his excitement, to tolerate frustrations, to organise himself and enjoy an activity, as he used to. Instead, he goes from expressions of distress to abrupt and unpredictable reactions, which are extreme enough to put his physical safety at risk. This situation lasted for many months. Like all young children, Teo depends on his parents to sustain his process of change and evolution, and when they fail to fulfil the structuring function, negative effects are generated in his fragile psychic functioning. Although he managed to make use of representational resources he had acquired throughout the analytic process and was able to express his sad feelings in words, the changes in his family situation and, above all, his parents' handling of it were effectively an attack on his fragile ego-integration. With his limited resources, Teo insistently affirms that "Dad is not here, Dad is never here". Could this be a way of decrying a symbolic place that his father has been unable to sustain and which is represented by returning to his mother's house and his childhood bedroom, which he now shares with his son, the two of them on a par, as equals, erasing the generation gap?

Throughout the analytical work, Teo has shown possibilities for change and the acquisition of ego resources to process and communicate his emotional experiences. However, the impact of the intersubjective on the bond with his parents hinders his incipient process of psychic structuring. The actual presence of parents in the analysis of the young child with a severe disorder also involves the weight of their personal histories and their own conflicts. These sometimes risk becoming disruptive and invading the child's analytical space, generating unpredictable effects that threaten the child's development.

References

Álvarez, A. (2020). A propósito del elemento de déficit en niños con autismo: psicoterapia basada en el psicoanálisis y factores del desarrollo [On the deficit element in children with autism: Psychotherapy based on psychoanalysis and developmental factors]. *eipea Magazine*, (9), 8–18. Heinemann, London.

Armesto, M., Zimerman, A., Ekboir, A. and Sahovaler, J. (2017). The multiple transferential field in child psychoanalysis. *Journal of Psychoanalysis*, 74(3), 103–112; ISSN: 0034-8740.

Bleichmar, S. (1984 [1986, 2008]). *En los orígenes del sujeto psíquico [On the origins of the psychic subject]*. Buenos Aires: Paidós.

Bleichmar, S. and Sigal de Rosenberg, A. M. (1995). *The place of parents in child psychoanalysis*. Buenos Aires: Lugar Editorial.

Brazelton, T., Koslowski, B. and Main, M. (1974). Origins of reciprocity. In M. Lewis and L. Rosenblum (Eds.). *Mother infant interaction*. New York: Wiley, pp. 57–70.

Bush de Ahumada, L. and Ahumada, J. (2015). *Contactando al niño autista. Cinco intervenciones psicoanalíticas tempranas exitosas [Contacting the autistic child. Five successful early psychoanalytic interventions]*. Buenos Aires: Ed. Biebel.

Cecchi, V. (2013). Algunas consideraciones acerca del autismo. [Some considerations about autism]. In *Autism clinics: Controversies. Controversies in Child and Adolescent Psychoanalysis. Journal*, (13), 59–64. Buenos Aires Psychoanal. Association.

Cecchi, V. (2021). *El psicoanálisis cura a los niños autistas con sus familias [Psychoanalysis heals autistic children with their families]*. Buenos Aires: Ed. Lumen.

Dolto, F. (1973). *La primera entrevista con el psicoanalista [The first interview with the psychoanalyst]*. Buenos Aires: Ed. Granica. London: Ed. Butterworth-Heinemann.

Freud, S. (1909). *Analysis of a fobia in a five-year-old boy* (Vol. X, Standard ed.). London: Hogardt Press.

Gergely, G. and Watson, J. S. (1996). The social biofeedback theory of parental affect-mirroring: The development of emotional self-awareness and self-control in infancy. *The International Journal of Psychoanalysis*, 77(6), 1181–1212.

Joyce, A. (2010). Discussion of Jorge L Ahumada and Luisa Busch de Ahumada's paper. In M.Leuzinger-Bohleber, J.Canestri and M.Target (Eds.). *Early development and its disturbances*. London: Karnac, pp. 175–183.

Klein, M. (1932). *The psychoanalysis of children*. Buenos Aires: Ed. W. W. Norton & Co.

Mannoni, M. (1976). *El niño su enfermedad y los otros [The child, his illness and the others]*. Buenos Aires: Ediciones Nueva Visión.

Meltzer, D. (1967). *The psycho-analytical process*. London: Ed. Butterworth-Heinemann.

Stern, D. (1985). *The interactional world of the infant: A view from psychoanalysis and developmental psychology*. New York: Basic Books.

Tronick, E. Z. (2007). Interactive mismatch and repair: Challenges to the coping infant. In E. Z. Tronick (Ed.). *The neurobehavioral and social-emotional development of infants and children*. New York: Norton & Co, pp. 155–163.

Winnicott, D. (1945). Primitive emotional development. *The International Journal of Psychoanalysis*, 26, 137–143. Laia, 1981.

Winnicott, D. (1960 [1965]). The theory of the parent-child relationship. In *The maturational processes and the facilitating environment London: The international psychoanalytical library* (Vol. 64). London: The Hogarth Press and the Institute of Psychoanalysis, pp. 1–276.

Winnicott, D. (1962). Dependence in infant care, in childcare and in the psychoanalytic setting. *The International Journal of Psychoanalysis*, 44, 339–344.

Zusman de Arbiser, S. (2009). Psicoanálisis infantil. Ayer y Hoy [Child psychoanalysis. Yesterday and today]. *Rev. De Psicoanálisis*, LXVI(2), 461–485.

7 The end of the psychoanalytical process of a child presenting with a serious disorder in early childhood

Ending the psychoanalytic process for a child presenting at the clinic with severe pathology in early childhood is a topic worthy of reflection. Given the extent of the difficulties presented by these patients, the question first arises as to our expectations and limitations in engaging in psychoanalytic therapy with them. I shall attempt to address this issue on the basis of the clinical account and in dialogue with leading authors.

Freud (1932) points out that the intention of psychoanalytic treatment is "to strengthen the ego . . . to widen its field of perception and enlarge its organisation, so that it can appropriate fresh portions of the id". "Where id was, there ego shall be", he adds (p. 72). In view of these considerations, I wonder whether the intention of the analytical process of the young child with autistic spectrum disorder differs in any way? Or rather, can the intention of the treatment be considered to be the same, even if the obstacles that arise are greater from the outset? I am inclined towards the latter alternative. In other words, I consider that the analysis of the patients in question shares the same intention as for any other analytic process. That is, to acquire resources to strengthen the ego and to master drive impulses. Or in Winnicott's terms (1958, p. 37), to generate the conditions so that the ego is strengthened by the impulses of the id.

However, when the origins of psychic functioning are at stake, as is the case for the children to whom I am referring, the possibility of strengthening the ego necessarily implies and is a condition for a work of psychic structuring and subjectivation. In addition, early failures in these patients' psychic structuring affect the development of ego functions, which may generate lasting effects that require specialised approaches. In some cases, difficulties in verbal language and/or motor skills interfere with the child's ability to communicate and learn, regardless of their willingness to interact and interest in learning. This disadvantage in the operational tools necessary for development generates frustration in the patient and can lead to the inhibition of functions and negative self-perception. This builds a complex scenario. What then are the conditions for ending the analytical treatment of these children?

DOI: 10.4324/9781032614823-9

To try and answer this question, I shall take as a starting point Melanie Klein's proposal in relation to all child analysis. According to this author, at the end of the analysis, it is hoped that as well as having the possibility of playing and working through traumatic situations, the child will be able to re-establish harmonious coexistence with his environment and his parents (1932). In this way, the expectations about the patient's evolution are based on two dimensions of experience, which are closely interrelated: the intrapsychic dynamics and the intersubjective scenario.

I shall address these aspects in the patients at hand and in the context of ending the analytic work. Finally, I shall refer to the child's own expressions that show he is aware of his or her own change process, which herald the end of the treatment.

Intrapsychic dynamics at the end of the analytic process: infantile neurosis

The acquisition of representational and symbolic resources, which along with increasing ego organisation enable playful activity and creative capacity, is a central element in the analytical process of young children with a severe disorder. This issue has been addressed in previous chapters, in which examples were provided from clinical material and reference was made to the first encounters with the child and parents or to the initial stages of treatment, so I do not intend to return to this aspect at this point.

Instead, my aim is to refer to a series of transformations in the content of fantasies, which each child manifested in his or her own unique way, and which evidenced a new and more complex form of psychic organisation. I refer in this way to infantile psychosexual development, understood in Freudian terms (Freud, 1905, 1916), and more precisely to infantile neurosis as the organising structure of intrapsychic dynamics regarding the oedipal conflict, with its fantasies, anguish and anxieties (Laplanche and Pontalis, 1968). As Ungar (2004, p. 20) points out, entry into this oedipal structure is achieved through analysis, which contributes to the subjectivation process of the child who presented a severe pathology.

The following brief snippets of clinical material from patients to whom I have already referred illustrate their vicissitudes and resources in accessing this new scenario.

Sexual differences and castration fantasy: "Damned pink"

After the first year of treatment, Matilde (Chapter 1), almost 4 and a half years old, draws two human figures on the blackboard, which she decides will be a girl and a boy.

M: Can you draw the girl for me? The girl's name is Ana. No, better Juan.
A: A girl called Juan?
M: "Yes, it's a girl's name, not a boy's name. It's a very pretty name," she says with false naturalness, as she colours in the boy. "Can you colour

in the girl for me? The boy was 2 years old, because the girl is older. The girl was 7 years old. She's missing something." She pauses contemplatively, looking at the figure of the girl and the boy in turn.

M: "I know!" She adds a detail to the drawing of the girl. "I've finished! A topknot!" She looks at me with satisfaction.

She then draws a flower in the girl's belly. This image reminds me of other drawings Matilde made during previous sessions, in which she had drawn babies instead of flowers in the bellies of human figures that she identified as "mummies".

M: Looking at me, she says, "No, she doesn't have a flower inside her belly," with special emphasis on the word "inside".

A: "Inside her belly?" I say, with the same emphasis. "Maybe when the girl is as big as a mummy, she can have babies inside her belly. Daddies don't, as you were saying the other time. But dads do have something that's missing in girls and mummies, don't they?" I say, somewhat knowingly.

M: "Ah! But that's different!" she says, rather annoyed.

A: "Yes, it is different. And you're telling me about these differences between girls and boys, between mummies and daddies."

M: "Now I need the colours. There are ten of them." She picks up the markers and counts them. "I'm counting them to make sure none are missing. Very good. I'll colour it in!" She carefully colours in the flower, and then adds a stem, which she especially highlights.

A: "With a stick?"

M: "I don't know, it's for the flower." She looks at me mischievously and laughs before adding, "No! She hasn't got a willy!!"

She continues vigorously making strokes on the stem, so the drawing becomes an ill-defined scribble. She tries to fix it by going over it with the marker, but a hole appears in the paper.

M: "Oops! It disappeared, and he was left with one eye!" She laughs anxiously. "You know? There was a banana in a shoe!" she laughs.

A: "You seem to be trying to think about these differences between girls and boys, between mummies and daddies, and what that's all about."

M: "I dropped my tail! I had a poo!" interrupts Matilde, raising her voice and laughing anxiously.

A: "Maybe sometimes it occurs to you that you once had a willy, like little boys, and that you dropped it like a poo!?"

M: "Yes, it fell off like a banana, like a stick – willy, like a willy that was skipping rope!" She laughs, saying these words quickly and anxiously, as she picks up the pink marker to colour in the girl. Looking at the marker, she adds, "Go on, give it to her! Silly pink! Damned pink!!" She laughs anxiously and repeats "damned pink!!"

A: "Is it damned to be a girl?"

Matilde looks at the markers on the table and shouts at them: "Damn you!!" She then fits four markers together lengthwise, so that the lids of the markers are joined to the ends of the others, forming a long row.

M: "Look at this! And they don't fall down!" she says, picking up the joined markers and holding them up in the air: "Look! It's a sword!" she adds triumphantly. Suddenly, one of them breaks off and falls. "Whoops! A little sword," she says, disappointed, "and the sword is cut. No, it's not cut." She tries to put the markers together again and reassemble the sword.

Having achieved a representation of herself as a subject with a sexual body, Matilde showed she was curious and interested in anatomical differences. In an attempt at elaboration, she deploys a series of representations that invoke a phallic-castrated opposition. The castration fantasy arose in her as a source of anguish and anxiety (Freud, 1908, 1923). *"Silly pink"*, *"Damned pink"*, she says, alluding to a colour that was culturally associated with femininity and that she herself associates with a "girl's" colour (Chapter 1). Between the acceptance or non-acceptance of the difference and *"the lack"*, the path towards the search for the father opened up, in an oedipal context.

Oedipal rivalry: "Being the king-daddy"

Fabian, aged 5 (Chapter 4), asks me to draw a castle on the blackboard. He then says something which I cannot understand, due to his significant difficulties in articulating, and I tell him this. He uses gestures and movements to represent something, and I understand that he is referring to a dragon. Fabian confirms this, and I draw one on the blackboard. He adds red eyes and sharp teeth. He points to a tower in the drawing of the castle and says "girl", so that I draw one.

A: "A girl in the castle? Is she perhaps a princess?" I ask, drawing the figure.

F: "Aha," he replies, nodding mischievously.

He looks at the drawing of the princess-girl and points to himself: "Mih," he says, while pointing to a place on the blackboard, and gesturing to show strength and a struggle.

I draw him fighting the dragon, as he asks me to. We look at the drawing together.

A: "Huh! How strong you are! You are fighting the dragon that keeps the princess imprisoned!"

He nods, looking proud and smiling.

A: "And what's the princess' name? Does she have a name?"

F: "Mummy!" he says, as if the answer were obvious.

A: "What? That can't be right!" I say, making an exaggerated gesture of bewilderment. "Mummy is the queen!" I add. "It can't be Mummy!"

F: "Let Mummy see this," he says. "This is not Daddy, this is 'mih'! And this is Mummy!" he adds, pointing to both characters on the board.

A: "Ah! You want to be the king-daddy!"

Despite his significant difficulties in expressing himself verbally due to a severe language disorder, in the course of the analytical process Fabián has gained resources to represent and elaborate his fantasies and conflicts in the dimension of play. In this vignette he portrays himself with the characteristics of strength and confronting the dragon-daddy who has trapped the princess-mummy. Thus, the rivalry with his father which is typical of the oedipal stage (Freud, 1912–1913) unfolds, evidencing an important evolution in his psychosexual development.

On origins: "And how are babies born?"

At the age of 6, Darius (Chapter 5) is in the first year of primary school. His interests have been widening. The characters of "elephant and tiger children" that arose in previous sessions continue to make appearances in playful scenes that he comes up with, demonstrating new and more complex abilities, to the delight of his parents. At this stage, Darius arrives at the sessions in good spirits and very willing. He writes the names of his friends and cousins and enjoys playing spelling games on the whiteboard. "I can do it on my own," he sometimes says, or when he finds himself in difficulties, he does not hesitate to ask for my help.

In one session during this period, he brings a leaflet which he tries to read but is unable to do so, although he generally reads very well. He contemptuously says, "It's whatever!" I notice that he is having difficulty because the leaflet contains acronyms instead of words, and I tell him what it is about. I tell him that each letter represents a word. Darius quickly gets the idea, and then writes his initials and mine, saying that they look like acronyms. Happy with this new discovery, he suggests playing that we are both teachers and that we set tasks for the elephant and tiger children, who are our pupils. Then, playing the role of teacher, he assigns each character a sheet of paper, on which he writes each of their initials. I notice that they both share the letter of my surname, and I point it out to him. "It's like they are your children," he says.

In the context of this playful scene, in which both characters, which he is managing, are doing their schoolwork very well, Darius tells me about an animated film he saw the day before. It is about two child characters who are ogres. "They live in a swamp, and when they have a bath they get all dirty! Because they bath in the swamp!" he says, laughing and grasping the ambiguity of the situation. As he continues to write some letters, he tells me that these characters had children, and that the children appear in the film. At a certain point, he falls silent and stops his activity. He looks at me, ponders for a moment, and very seriously asks me, "Nahir, and how are babies born? Is it a secret?"

Darius shows curiosity and openness to new learning. He enjoys his investigations and his sense of humour. Growth on a realistic level, in other words accepting his limitations, is making headway against the illusion of infantile omnipotence. Asking for the analyst's help shows that he recognises and accepts the generational difference and realises that the adult has knowledge and experiences, which opens up the prospect in him of exploring them. He is thus keen to assimilate the concept of acronyms and creatively practices using his initials, mine and those of the characters in the improvised game. In this context, his question about how babies are born alludes to the sexuality of the parents. Darius immediately answers himself by mentioning "a secret". That is, of something private, to which he has no access. Thus, the boy's sexual curiosity coexists with intellectual interests that broaden and enrich his world of experiences. The complex and developed psychic mechanism of sublimation has allowed him access to culture.

The intersubjective scenario at the end of the analytical process

The child's acquisition of resources that create an interest in and openness towards a world of affective and social bonds is a key achievement in the analytical process of the patients in question. At the end of treatment, it is expected that the child will be able to deploy his or her growing intersubjective capacities in the settings where he or she lives, that is, in the family and school settings. As Winnicott puts it,

> In the analysis of young children the analyst is aided considerably by the tremendous changes that naturally take place in the 5, 6 or 7 year old child. As the early analysis draws to a close, the changes in question, undoubtedly made possible by the analysis, follow one after the other. Thus, any improvement brought about by analysis is augmented by the natural course of events.
>
> (Winnicott, 1958)

However, this possibility does not merely depend on the patient and his or her new resources but also involves the flexibility of the context: the child must be allowed to reposition itself in the intersubjective dynamics, in function of his or her gradual evolution. When these conditions are met, as Winnicott (1962) proposes, the child's home, relationships and friends carry out part of the treatment.

The following vignette illustrates some of these aspects of the parent-child bond. Later on, however, I shall discuss some of the complexities that may arise when the child starts school, with repercussions for his or her development.

Tiago and his father: "Did he tell you he's a champion?!"

At the age of 6 and after a long period of making up fantastic superhero stories in which phallic potency and oedipal rivalry were expressed, Tiago (Chapter 2) became interested in board games. He openly expresses his desire to win and is angry when he does not.

In one session, he discovers a box with the classic game of draughts, which is a strategy game. He tells me he's never seen it and asks me how to play. We read the rules together, and then we play. During the game I show him moves that would help him to win and moves that would not, and I do the same on my turn, taking into account my own possible moves. Tiago is very interested, and we continue to jointly think about possible moves for each other. At the end of the session, his father arrives to pick him up. Tiago runs out to meet him and asks him if he knows how to play draughts. "I learned today!" he tells him happily and proudly.

"I'm the world champion," replies the father, enthusiastically, adding, "I learned to play when I was your age."

"Do we have a draughts set at home?" asks Tiago.

"Do we have a draughts set?" his father says, thinking. "And if we don't have one, don't worry! I'm sure I can get one tomorrow," he says, with a knowing smile.

In the next session, Tiago resumes playing draughts. He tells me that he has been playing with his daddy, who has taught him other moves, and he shows them to me throughout the game. In the meantime, he tells me some stories his father told him about when he himself was a child. He says his father learned to play draughts with his father, in other words with Tiago's grandfather. He also mentions chess and invites me to play. He says that "it's an even more difficult game", but that his father knows how to play, and that he has taught him how.

At the end of the session, when I open the door, I see the father is very pleased. "Did he tell you he's a draughts and chess champion?" he says to me, referring to the boy.

Tiago smilingly clarifies: "I'm learning!"

I tell his father that Tiago invited me to play chess today and that he seems eager to learn.

"Yes," says his father, enthusiastically and with a certain sense of relief. "He's a champion, the way he is learning!"

"And also letters!" adds Tiago.

Set in the scenario of oedipal rivalry, Tiago measures his father's knowledge, asking him if he knows how to play draughts. He also tells him about his new learning: "*I learned today,*" he says, enthusiastically. He encounters a champion dad in his father's response: "*I am the world champion.*" At the same time, he offers himself as a role model with which to identify: "*I learned to play when I was your age.*" Appreciative of the child's interest, the father does not hesitate in his willingness to get the game and to share this playful scenario with Tiago, which is also a scenario of phallic competition. Thus, empowered by his father, Tiago reaffirms his position as a rival, perceiving himself as having the capacity and resources to enter into competition.

In the next session, the child reports that the father has provided him with new resources. He says he has taught him new moves, and also chess, a game he describes as "*even more difficult*". Then, the figure of the grandfather, who taught Tiago's father how to play, enters into this father-son encounter by way of mention. The boy is thus located in a generational chain of boys who receive valuable knowledge from their elders, which empowers them to become "champions".

At the end of the session, Tiago's father expresses his pleasure in seeing that his son is an intelligent child capable of learning. He's *"a champion,"* he says, as he had said about himself. In response, Tiago realistically expresses his limitations, along with an expectation of getting to know more: *"I'm learning,"* he says. In addition, he spontaneously and enthusiastically mentions that he is learning to write letters. He thus expresses his appreciation for acquiring intellectual and cultural elements of a symbolic world with a framework of shared rules.

Emma and her new school: "I did it! The teacher helped me, and I did it!"

Starting school presents a number of complexities for our group of the children. This is the setting where the resources that the patient has acquired during the analytical process are put to the test, and it involves the challenge of sharing a group space, in an exogamous context and with the objective of learning. For a child with fragilities in its subjective structuring, all this configures a scenario that can become intrusive and hostile, reactivating and accentuating any existing insecurities.

I believe that the flexibility of the school is a relevant element in enabling the child to continue the process of subjectivation and to strengthen the deployment of ego functions. This condition requires the school to have an individual view of the child, in dialogue with the treating professionals, with confidence in the child's capacities and tolerance of his or her developmental periods. While some patients do not require follow-up by a child psychiatrist or specific approaches for adequate language and/ or motor development, this is not the most frequent scenario. Early difficulties in the process of subjectivation often result in language dysfunctions or disorders of varying degrees, regardless of whether the child has acquired communicative intentionality and willingness to communicate during the analytical process. An example of this situation can be seen in the vignette of Fabian presented in this chapter. Motor difficulties may also persist, which become more evident in a school context where graphic representation is practiced and the child accesses the written word. These disadvantages in the tools necessary for verbal and written communication interfere with the child's social integration at school, and also with their learning.

Thus, when the school is inflexible and lacks openness, new difficulties arise, which make the patient and his or her parents more brittle, creating more suffering and a lack of hope. On these occasions, instead of being a starting point from which to address the situation, early diagnosis can mistakenly lead to a perspective that stigmatises the child, without giving rise to an expectation of development, or even impeding perceptions of the child's progress. At this point, a change of school can offer the child an opportunity to reposition themselves in the intersubjective dynamics and in their relationship with learning. Patients I have mentioned in previous chapters had to take this path. The following is an account of the vicissitudes and experiences of a young girl in this situation.

Emma came to the clinic at the age of 2 years and 10 months with a diagnosis of autistic spectrum disorder. From the first months of sessions three times a week, she showed a favourable evolution, which her parents noticed in the home environment. She showed signs of interaction, gradually developed some elementary play activities, and her vocabulary was expanding. Some time later, she began to mention herself in the first person "I". However, at the end of the school year, her teachers gave a very negative assessment of the child and her abilities. Her parents were discouraged. They were left with a lot of unresolved questions and decided to change schools.

At almost 4 years old, and shortly after the start of the school year, Emma began speech therapy and psychomotor therapy, in accordance with the approach and norms of the new educational institution. These professionals noted that both functions seemed to be lowered in pragmatic terms but did not hesitate in describing Emma as a capable, receptive and resourceful learner. However, at the school Emma was seen as a "different" child, and the suggestions made towards her only isolated her. Her parents were becoming increasingly discouraged. Their frustrations and distress interfered with the bond with their child. At my request, and in consultation with the other treating professionals, Emma's parents began dubiously and cautiously searching for a new school again.

At the age of 5, and a few months after the start of the school year at her third school, the child asks me to come in for a session with her mother. Although it was unusual for her during that period of the analytic process, I accept her proposal. The mother sits down in an armchair. Emma climbs onto the couch and does a somersault. "I did it!" she exclaims happily. "The teacher helped me, and I did it! At the other place I couldn't do it, and my knees hurt" she adds, referring to her previous school. Her mother looks at me and nods with a sad expression on her face. "It's true, she's learned to do a somersault," she says. I notice that Emma is calmer, and I mention this to her mother. "Since she left the other school, she no longer sucks her thumb or bites her nails," she says. "The other day, she told me about the other school for the first time. She said a girl told her that her drawings were ugly and that she told the other children not to be friends with her. She was very upset when she told me that, and she started to cry. I hugged her. She never told me anything. She was having a hard time," she adds, sadly.

Emma remains silent, listening attentively, and looks at me. I tell her that it all must have been very difficult for her and that Mummy and Daddy saw that she was having a hard time and that's why they found this new school, where they help children to learn and have friends. She nods, very seriously. She mentions the name of "a friend from the new school" and that of her teacher. She also says that when she arrives at the school she sees "the big children from the high school" and "the babies", who "go to other houses", she adds, referring to the buildings that house the different sectors. The mother listens to her and nods, reaffirming what she is saying.

At the next session, she again asks to go in with her mother. She draws two figures on the blackboard, which she identifies as "Mummy and Daddy". This is the first time I have seen her drawing spontaneously and with commitment. Adding a shorter figure in the middle, she says, "And this is me." All three figures have a smile on their faces. She writes the number "5", saying that this is her age, and then she also writes the number "6", saying that this is how old she is going to be. Finally, she writes her name, "Mummy" and "Daddy". I am surprised. Until now, she had never written or shown any interest in letters or numbers. She then invites her mother to play. She suggests making a building with blocks. She creates a scene with familiar characters and situations. The two of them play, smiling and talking to each other all the time. For the first time I notice that the mother is relieved and enjoying the encounter with her daughter. I tell Emma that she is showing me they are all happier and calmer at home now and that she and Mummy have a great time playing together.

I also refer to Emma's development, her interest and willingness to draw and write letters and numbers, and the perception of herself growing and learning. The mother is moved and says, "Now she is happy to go to school. Seeing her happy gives us a lot of hope."

Historicisation of the analytical process

Up to this point, the conditions for the completion of the analytic process of the children in question have been explored on the basis of the development of intrapsychic dynamics and of the resources available for the intersubjective scenario. Along with this, a new element to be expected towards the end of treatment is the child's recognition of its own progress, with the capacity to historicise its change and growth process within the analytical bond. I shall illustrate these aspects on the basis of clinical material from two patients to whom I have already referred in previous chapters.

"I'm going my own way!"

Javier (Chapter 2) has been evolving well, and almost four years after the start of his treatment, on arriving for a session he reminds me that he is 6 and a half years old. Very happy, he says that he learned to ride a bicycle on his own without stabilisers, and that his parents applauded him. In the meantime, he picks up the ball, demonstrates his football skills, and pulling two chairs up against the wall as improvised goalposts, he asks me to shoot the ball, and he is going to save. He also tells me that his tackling has improved a lot. I note that this is true. Javier has a better command of his body and his movements; he is confident and enjoys physical activity and sport.

At one point, he remembers playing ball at his late grandmother's house. "When I remember, I'm afraid that my mother is going to die. Thinking about it makes me want to cry," he says, a little emotionally.

He then moves on to board games, which he refers to as "big children's games." "They are for 6-, 7- and 8-year-olds," he adds. He says he wants to learn, and asks me to explain the rules. We play various games together. Javier makes a scoreboard, on which he writes his name and mine, and the winner of each game gets a point.

In one of these games, a token must be moved around the board to reach the finish line. He rolls a higher score on the die, and so his token is placed ahead of mine.

J: "I'm leaving you behind, Nahir! I'm going my own way!" he says, smiling warmly and enjoying seeing himself as the winner of the game.

I tell him that it is true; today he is showing me that he can do a lot of big boy things and that he is very happy about that. I add that I also see that he has grown up a lot and that he can go his own way.

Referring to a sports competition at his school, he says that his team won "the gold medal in the championship".

Javier enjoys his new skills and abilities. He perceives his growth and shows curiosity and interest in learning. With spontaneity and the capacity to enjoy his achievements, he displays a wide range of affects during the session, including the transferential allusion to the loss of a significant figure.

In the next session, he chooses a board game once more. He wins again and expresses how pleased he is. At a certain point, he goes under the couch to look for a token that had fallen down, and I notice that he takes a few moments.

A: "What happened?" I ask him.
J: "It's like when I was a baby!" he replies, laughing and remembering what he used to do in the early days of our work together.

As he is leaving, he asks me how much longer he is going to be coming. I tell him that I have also been wondering about this for some time. I add that I would like to talk to his parents and then see how long we can carry on working together. Javier accepts and suggests playing with a car he used to play with in the early days. We both sat on the floor, close to each other. As we play, he starts a conversation.

J: "Do you remember when we used to play with this?" he asks, talking about the car.
A: "Yes, you were little. It was almost at the beginning."
J: "And are you going to remember everything?" he asks me, a little emotionally.
A: "I'll remember you and probably also a lot of the things we played together."
J: "I'm not going to see you anymore," he says, looking sad. He remains silent, and then, in a warm and thoughtful tone, he asks, "and will other children come?"
A: "Hmm, and what do you think?"
J: "I want them to," he affirms.
A: "You want them to? And why is that?"

Javier looks at me affectionately. He doesn't seem to know how to explain it.

A: "Maybe you want other children to be able to get things that help them grow up, like you felt you got here?"
Javier nods. He is touched. The session takes on a poignant atmosphere.

J: "Can you tell me about the first day I came?"

A: "Yes." I tell him about the first interview he came to with his father. He looks at me, listens attentively and asks for details. He smiles tenderly. He is moved, and I too find it moving to remember those first meetings, as I see him grown up, expressive and affectionate.
      "Let's play a big boy's game," he then proposes. He chooses a card game, which is a game of luck and strategy. I help him to win the game, giving him some hints on how to succeed.

J: "I won! I won! I won!" he chants happily.

A: "Of course you won! You gained many things in this work together, and it is very important for you to go away a winner, because to think about saying goodbye, as we did today, is also to lose this space, which has been so important in helping you to grow and to have friends.
      We collected up the material to say goodbye. When he hears his mother ringing the doorbell, Javier immediately says, "I'm going under the couch!" and again he gets under the couch.

A: "Again, like when you were little!" I say, friendly and smiling.

J: "I came in here forever," he says with a smile.
      Then he runs off to meet his mother. He hugs her warmly and tells her that we were "talking about stopping coming". "We are very pleased," his mother says. "And you should see how well he speaks French!"

With the option of finalising the analysis established, Javier invites me to reminisce about our early encounters. Against the backdrop of the transferential bond, we create a history of his analytical process by means of his games and questions. It is also his history of change and development, from *"when he was a baby"* to the *"big children's game"*.

"And that was the end of the story"

Darius (Chapter 5), in a session that takes place in the middle of his first year of primary school, he comes in happy and willing, as he usually did at that stage. In recent months he had shown significant development. As in previous sessions, he suggests playing with the "elephant and tiger children" characters and their parents. He says that the children "are building a turbo plane" and "a mobile home", which he builds out of blocks. As usual, the parents, whose role I am playing, are happy and proud of their children's skills. At a certain point, Darius stops, looks at me and, alluding to the box containing his playing material, asks me,

D: "What are you going to do with my box when I stop coming here?"
      I am surprised by his question. I tell him that we'll think about it together but that he's probably also wondering how long he's still going to be coming here.

D: "And why am I still coming here?" he asks me.

A: "You are still coming to help you grow up, to have friends, to do well at school."

D: "I have friends," he affirms, without hesitation.

A: "It's true, you have friends, and that's very nice. Now we have to try to make it so that you want to do the work at school that your teacher asks you to, because that will help you to learn more, and you will feel better."

D: "All the tasks?!" he exclaims, rather annoyed.

A: "Well, yes, just like your friends do, because you can!"

A few weeks later I have his parents come to my office. For the first time in years I see that they are happy and relaxed, even joking and celebrating Darius' mischievous attitudes, which they tell me about. They happily mention his recent birthday party with friends, his willingness in his everyday life at home and at school and even the complaints he makes to his parents when he feels he is being offered something meant for a small child. "In fact, it's all quiet at home," says his father, laughing and amazed at his own appreciation. "Now he wants to learn to play football, and he asks me the rules," he adds. We agreed that I would contact the school and the treating psychomotor therapist to find out how they saw the child's functioning. And if all went well, we would start working on terminating treatment. In the end, we continued working for a few more months until the end of the school year.

In one session during this period, Darius arrives and hides behind a large cushion. "You have to find me," he says. Then, laughing, he adds, "You won't find me anymore!"

A: "This time I'll find you. But it's true that I soon won't find you anymore, because in a while we're going to say goodbye. And then, I won't find you here anymore because you won't be coming."

Darius remains still and silent for a few moments. He comes out of hiding, stands in front of me and very seriously asks me, "Does that mean I'm not coming anymore?"

A: "Yes, as we have been discussing for a while. Now we are working on saying goodbye."

He opens his box of materials and, taking out a drawing, followed by others, each time asks me, "And what's this?"

I tell him what I remember about each drawing, and that it seems to me he wants to test my memory, as if he wants to know if I'm going to remember him and what we have worked on together.

D: "And why won't I be coming anymore?"

A: "Because you are growing up very well, you feel good at home, you have friends, you want to learn, and you can now do a lot of things that you like doing. So you don't need to come here like you did before. And that means we have done really good work."

Darius takes a little ball out of from his box that we had made together some time ago. It is the representation of a ball belonging to an animated character, which has the power to evolve and give greater abilities to magical characters, who have powers.

A: "It's the magic ball, like the magic of you growing and developing here."

D: "I'm going to sleep under the desk!" he says, positioning himself curled up under the desk. "I'm playing that I'm camping. It seems I'm camping alone. No! I've spotted the other bed, Nahir! Lie down over there!" he says, pointing to the couch.

I do so. And from there, I say to him,

A: "Maybe you think you might feel lonely when we say goodbye?"

He invites me to come and sit next to him, under the desk, and says that one of the magical characters wants to trap us inside the little ball.

A: "Ugh, trapped! How horrible!" I say in an exaggerated tone. "You can't see your friends, or your mum and dad, or your teacher! That would be awful!"

D: "If we get trapped, we'll die!"

A: "Of course! To be trapped is like dying. It's not being able to move forward, and it's not good to be trapped coming here when you can already do so many things that you like doing and continue growing."

At the next session, he arrives wearing his football team's shirt, which is also his father's and grandfather's. He suggests we play memory games and wins several times. He then tells me that he is going on a school camp, so he won't be able to come "next time".

D: "Mateo is going to the camp, and he behaved badly. He pulled Juan, and I defended him," he explains, "because the teacher says that they are all friends, but I was furious with Mateo, because he pulled Juan, and I hit him with the bag I had in my hand to make him let go. It was my snack bag, and they took me to the head teacher, because Mateo got hurt. But he pulled Juan," he adds, very seriously.

D: "And there is another boy who also behaves badly. He doesn't finish his work! He just writes the title!" he says dismissively and very expressively.

A: "Well, maybe that boy needs help to finish his work."

D: "No, no, he behaves badly," he adds, with conviction and shaking his head. "At the start of first year I misbehaved too. I don't know why. And I didn't do my work. Not now. Now I do it, and I behave myself."

A: "That's nice. Those are very important changes. I'm sure they make you feel better."

Darius nods and accepts my words with a proud expression.

For several months we worked on our farewell, which took place at the end of the school year. He arrives at the last session excited. He gives me a beautiful gift that he says he bought for me with his parents. He goes to the whiteboard and writes, "Nahir and . . ." He looks at me expectantly. I write his name in the ellipses. I also mention our work together, which is ending today, which will leave us with many memories of Nahir and Darius, I add, reading our names on the whiteboard.

He draws a sad face and, next to it, a happy face. I refer to the sadness of our saying goodbye and also to the happiness at what we have both achieved to reach this moment. Darius looks at me and nods. He then starts to build something with blocks, as he had usually done of late. I remain seated on the floor next to him and watch him working as we talk.

D: "It's a spaceship, with protective windows and alarms, and also these barriers," he tells me.

A: "I see it has quite a lot of protection."

D: "These are security cameras. If it rains, it will have a protective roof to protect it from the rain. It's the sturdiest spaceship, because there are protective windows," he says, while adding blocks. He builds something very elaborate. "The spaceship used to be explosive. This is another deck," he says, "like we used to do before."

A: "How nice! How well you remember what we built together! You felt very protected here. And you know that if there is an alarm or if you want to come and tell me something or visit me at any time, you tell your mum and dad and you will be able to do that."

D: "I know. I know that," he says seriously. Then, looking at his spaceship, he asks, "How does it look? Beautiful!" he replies, proudly.

A: "Maybe you feel that this path here helped you to build beautiful things that make you feel good and stronger. Sturdier, like the space-ship. I also see it like that."

D: There it is. This is the roof. It's like a spaceship that I built. Because, do you know what this spaceship was before?" he asks me with an air of suspense, looking at me as I look at him, intrigued. "We're imagining that someone else built it before, but it broke, and we're putting it back together. Look what I put on it, because if something happens to it, it'll have these protective roofs for rain, storm, accidents. If there's a strong wind, we don't want it to blow away. The new spaceship is on its way."

A: "Well, let's hope that there aren't any accidents, and that it doesn't get into any difficulties. We have worked very well to make you feel safe and secure. I am sure that things are going to go well."

D: "That's why we're making a new spaceship, because the other one was weak."

A: "You are also stronger now as you say goodbye, like the spaceship."
I tell him it is time for his father to come and pick him up.

D: "And it's over! The end of the story is over," he says, finishing his con-struction and looking at me with an affectionate smile.
As we say goodbye, he wants to leave the spaceship assembled. He puts the "elephant and tiger sons" characters inside it. Could this be the expression of a fantasy of remaining in the analytical space?

As we say our farewells, Darius expresses his sadness, his happiness and also his fears. Identified with the analytical function, he compares his past and present self, showing that he perceives his change and development.

The *"new spaceship"* that he builds, and which represents him, reaffirms his expression of these experiences. His parting expression is ambiguous. Is the story over? Or has the ending been eliminated, resulting in an open-ended, never-ending story?

In the analytic work with Darius and other children, the hope is that the traces of a transferential bond will remain (forever?), which allows them to continue their development process, generating new stories with others, with greater confidence in their resources in the face of the challenges and joys of growing up.

References

Freud, S. (1905). *Three essays on the theory of sexuality* (Vol. VII, Standard ed.). London: Hogarth Press, pp. 123–246.

Freud, S. (1908). *Infantile sexuality* (Vol. VII, Standard ed.). London: Hogarth Press, pp. 173–206.

Freud, S. (1912–1913). *Totem and taboo. Standard edition of complete works* (Vol. XIII). London: Hogarth Press.

Freud, S. (1916). Libidinal development and sexual organisation. In *Introductory lectures on psychoanalysis* (No. 21). Standard Edition of complete works (Vol. XVI). London: Hogarth Press.

Freud, S. (1923). *The infantile genital organisation. Standard Edition of complete works* (Vol. XXIII). London: Hogarth Press.

Freud, S. (1932). *New introductory lectures on psychoanalysis* (No. 31). Standard Edition of complete works (Vol. XXII). London: Hogarth Press.

Klein, M. (1932). *The psychoanalysis of children.* Buenos Aires: Ed. W. W. Norton & Co.

Laplanche, J. and Pontalis, J. B. (1988 [1973]). *The language of psychoanalysis.* London: Karnac Books.

Ungar, V. (2004, March). La neurosis infantil como un organizador del desarrollo [Childhood neurosis as a developmental organiser]. *Revista Brasileira de Psicoterapia, 5*(2).

Winnicott, D. (1958 [1965]). The capacity to be alone. In *The maturational processes and the facilitating environment.* London: Karnac Books, pp. 29–36.

Winnicott, D. (1962). Dependence in infant care, in childcare and in the psycho-analytic setting. *The International Journal of Psycho-Analysis, 44,* 339–344.

Part II

Psychoanalysis and community

Contributions to an interdisciplinary approach to risk detection and promotion of early emotional development

To Dr Mónica Oliver,
dear friend and colleague.
In memoriam.

8 The paediatric well-baby visit

An opportunity for infant mental health care

From this chapter onwards, psychoanalytic contributions about early emotional development (Winnicott, 1960) are transposed to an operational level to generate a dialogue with the professionals closest to the infant and his or her parents, to the benefit of infant mental health care and promotion.

Various psychoanalytic theories indicate the significance of early intersubjective experiences underlying the mother-infant relationship for the process of subjectivation and the development of the newborn's potential capacities (Winnicott, 1960; Emde et al., 1976; Tronick et al., 1978; Stern, 1985; Lebovici, 1988a; Cramer, 1990; Fonagy et al., 2002; Benjamin and Atlas, 2015). At the same time, it is recognised that this intersubjective dynamic includes both the conscious and unconscious psychic and emotional life of the mother (Lebovici, 1988b; Cramer, 1990; Kreisler et al., 1997; Laplanche, 1989).

Furthermore, in the 1970s observations began on the micro-analytical study of videotaped interactions in the mother-infant dyad, allowing identification of the primary elements of communication in daily exchanges within the dyad which facilitate the infant's self-perception as having a psychic and emotional life, and recognition and regulation of his or her emotions, among other aspects (Gergely and Watson, 1996). In line with this, rhythm, mutuality and synchrony in verbal and non-verbal communications between mother and infant are identified as principles which organise psychic life and form the basis of psychic and emotional processes of greater complexity (Stern, 1985; Benjamin, 2002).

In recent decades, the infant has also been the subject of study within various disciplines. Psychiatrists, psychologists, paediatricians, anthropologists, sociologists, nutritionists, and more recently neuroscientists seek to identify factors that positively or negatively affect development. What these approaches all have in common is the notion that the first years of life are a key period for the subject's future. From then on, research in early childhood has been placed in a priority place for the prevention and promotion of children's health, as well as for the care of the development of the capacities of the individual and society as a whole (Heckman, 2015;

DOI: 10.4324/9781032614823-11

World Health Organization, 2015). Recent contributions from neuroscience recognise the dependence of the newborn on its milieu and concur that development cannot be envisaged in isolation from experience (Harvard University, 2014). This perspective identifies the infant's relationship with parental figures as a relevant dimension that exerts a lasting influence on structural and functional aspects of child development (Fox et al., 2010; Worthman et al., 2016; Harvard University, 2014).

This confluence of scientific knowledge shared by different disciplines presents an opportunity for psychoanalysis to offer outreach work in the community, contributing to the care of early relationships and infantile emotional development. To this end, the following chapters describe and analyse different elements of a work project that originated in 2006 in socially highly vulnerable public health centres in the metropolitan area of Montevideo, the capital city of Uruguay, and which has since gained acceptance and been expanded to different settings and regions. In this initiative, psychoanalysis takes on the challenge of leaving its traditional clinical setting to actively go out and meet the infant, its parents and the practitioners most involved in attending and caring for it, strengthening the resources of paediatricians, family doctors and other members of the health team, in order to take a preventive approach to early emotional development and infant mental health, starting at the primary care level.

This psychoanalytic intervention in the community is based on the idea that, as Bleichmar (1995) affirms, the formative reality of the child's psyche involves not only parental functions but also the substitutes for the original objects, which include health and education practitioners. In 2019, this work received recognition in the form of a Psychoanalysis in the Community Health Area award and is in line with the current strategy of the International Psychoanalytic Association (IPA) to offer resources and tools from our discipline for the benefit of the society in which we find ourselves.

This initiative considers the regular well-baby visit as a universal instance for the care of the newborn's potential capacities, while recognising the paediatrician and family doctor who perform paediatric check-ups as the practitioners closest to the infant and his or her parents, and thus have greater opportunities for early detection of any risks in infant development. Moreover, the profound changes that occur in the woman's psyche on experiencing motherhood and the transference mode that she consequently establishes with the health practitioner who takes care of the infant's health (Stern, 1995) are considered factors which make the paediatric check-up a potential scenario to foment maternal sensitivity and her capacity to care for and relate to her infant.

The work presented in the following chapters was conducted in the real-life setting of clinical practice, using the methodology of action research (Lewin, 1946), while its results which benefitted practitioners, the infant and her parents were evaluated according to rigorous parameters shared by different disciplines. It is a model of infant care during the well-baby visit which can be replicated by other practitioners in different regions and health centres.

This proposal aims to be a psychoanalytic contribution for the creation of primary prevention programmes and promotion of emotional develop-ment and infant mental health in the framework of public policies for the benefit of citizens, in particular disadvantaged populations, in accordance with the objectives set out by the World Health Organisation (2015) for its 2016–2030 strategy.

The mother's psyche and transference dynamic in the well-baby visit

In recent years, scientific studies have identified modifications which favour sensitivity occurring in the maternal brain structure during the peri-natal period. These are activated by inferring the intentions, thoughts and needs of the other (Barba-Müller, 2015; Barba-Müller et al., 2018). Far from contradicting psychoanalytical tenets, these findings are the biological cor-relate to the clinical insights of a long tradition of psychoanalysts who have been working with mother-baby dyads for several decades.

Winnicott (1956) highlights from his experience as a paediatrician and psychoanalyst the mother's heightened sensitivity concerning the birth of the infant, which allows her to recognise its needs and adapt to them through experiences connected with empathy and identification (1960). These conditions are taken up by Stern (1995) from his clinical experience in psychotherapeutic interventions on early bonding. This author stresses that the mother undergoes an important psychic reorganisation during this phase of life, with profound changes in her identity as a daughter and a mother. He describes a series of experiences that include fears and anxie-ties in relation to her maternal capacity to sustain the life and development of her infant, as well as the need and search for a supporting matrix or network comprising reference figures who allow her to feel *"accompanied, valued, appreciated, instructed and aided"* in her maternal role (p. 177).

Stern emphasises to clinicians the importance of taking into account the affective intensity of the mother's fear that she will be unable to provide adequate care and points out that these experiences, along with the impor-tant need to feel recognised and reaffirmed in her maternal role, condition a particular transference dynamic in relation to the practitioner. He adds that these experiences and needs predispose the mother towards an encounter with an active, emotionally involved practitioner who is able to recognise her capacity to provide care and attention to the infant. Conversely, this author highlights that the mother is extremely susceptible to any com-ments the practitioner makes about the infant, which she may perceive as a disqualification or a questioning of her capacity as a mother. According to Stern, these experiences of vulnerability and sensitivity also mean that the therapeutic alliance with the practitioner, once established, continues to act in the mother's psyche even when the doctor is not physically present. In this sense, the author argues that the transference relationship with the practitioner potentially becomes a sustaining force of help and support for the mother and her capacities. According to these contributions, these are the most sensitive elements that need to be taken into account in any clinical situation at this stage in a woman's life.

The work presented in the next section assumes that these maternal experiences and expectations transcend the therapeutic space of the dyad, instead having implications for the bond that the mother establishes with any practitioner who provides care to the infant, especially within a sustained framework of continuity of care. With these aspects in mind, this initiative proposes that each member of the health team can become a valuable influence on the mother's mental capacity to care for and relate to her infant, the practitioner's sensitivity being the determining factor for this.

In this way, in a context of a mother's profound psychic reorganisation and openness towards new identifying references that reaffirm her in her maternal function, and with a special sensitivity with which she empathetically experiences the care that the practitioner provides for the infant (Stern, 1995), the well-baby visit with its transferential component indirectly creates a potential change scenario for the maternal capacity, and in her experience of feeling recognised and valued.

From this perspective, the work presented in the following chapters attempts to explore the greater potential of existing societal resources, taking the scenario of daily interactions between the health team, infants and their parents as an opportunity to promote a healthy relational setting which favours parental sensitivity to the experiences and needs of the infant, thus benefitting the early relationship.

Doctor-infant interaction as a setting for promoting early emotional development

Different models of psychoanalytic interventions in early bonding aim to directly or indirectly modify the parental mental representations which hinder interaction, although there are differences in methodology and the source of clinical information on which each approach focuses. Both Fraiberg (Fraiberg et al., 1975) and Lieberman (Lieberman and Paul, 1993) interpret the mother's mental representations in order to generate a change in the dynamics of early interaction, as do Cramer and Palacio-Espasa (1993), albeit from a different perspective.

In contrast, the starting point for another line of intervention is the infant's overt behaviour, in which the gestures, bodily movements and actions that the infant displays during the clinical situation take on the meaning of non-verbal or preverbal communications. In this regard, Lebovici and Weil-Harper (1995) point out that the observation of spontaneous and interactive behaviours of infants provides information on their development, motor skills and somatic expression, as manifestations of their psychological and emotional functioning. Winnicott (1941) also describes infant observation in a fixed setting during a paediatric visit as a resource that gives us an insight into key aspects of the child's emotional development and a basis from which to carry out therapeutic work. Reaffirming this idea, Stern (1995) highlights the important impact that specific and limited observations on the infant's functioning can have on the mother and points out that it is her emotional state which enables this effect. He maintains that "the important point is that the mother's representations of her infant can be radically altered by placing the clinical focus exclusively on the infant's overt behaviour" (pp. 130, 131).

Infant observation is also a methodological resource in paediatrics, especially when it is carried out in a standardised procedure or within a specific framework. Brazelton (1978, 1994) is one of the main references in this regard. He focuses on observation of the infant's overt behaviour during the paediatric examination to point out to the parents the child's capabilities and interest in the relationship and the need to modulate stimuli to foster interaction. This model of intervention enables parents to change their perception of their infant by discovering new capacities in him or her. At the same time, incorporating new ways of relating boosts the parents' confidence in their resources, which benefits their self-perception (Domínguez et al., 2009). Some authors (Keefer et al., 2009) refer to the use of this observation model in routine paediatric check-ups to facilitate emotional bonding between parents and infants, while others (Nugent, 2015) suggest using it during the first few months of an infant's life to sensitise parents to the newborn's communication skills.

In relation to the previous statements, infant observation is an area of shared interest in the work presented in the following chapters, facilitating dialogue between paediatrics and psychoanalytic contributions, to the benefit of infant mental health care. To this end, the infant's overt behaviour when interacting with the doctor during the paediatric check-up forms the starting point for an approach towards early detection of risk and promotion of early emotional development. This approach is based on a psychoanalytic perspective, which recognises that interactions are anchored in a representational dimension.

This initiative assumes that one relevant aspect of the paediatric check-up is the attitude of the practitioner carrying it out. As Leblanc and Soulé (1995) point out, no action of caregiving in connection with vital human needs can be detached from the person providing it: the vocation to serve is a commitment of the practitioner as a person, with her own psycho-emotional characteristics. In this sense, the emotional commitment of the practitioner towards the infant during clinical practice is an indispensable condition to enable a vision of the infant as an experiencing subject, with a psychic and emotional life, rather than considering him or her to merely be an object of care.

Based on this concept, this work proposes a training programme for practitioners who provide care to infants and their parents, based on an interdisciplinary perspective of the emotional needs of the dyad and the importance of interactions for healthy emotional development. Furthermore, it includes a standardised and internationally validated infant observation guide for early detection of key risk indicators in early emotional development, such as infant withdrawal (Escala Alarme Détresse Bébé, Guedeney and Fermanian, 2001). Certain complementary resources from psychoanalytic work in early bonding and with young children are also presented. These, adapted to the setting of the paediatric check-up, broaden the practitioner's tools when communicating with the infant and also with the parents.

These resources comprise different technical modalities, such as verbalisation by the practitioner of the emotional initiatives and expressions perceived in the infant, assigning them intentionality or meaning (Fonagy et al., 2002) and "theatrical" verbalisation of these aspects (Stern, 1995) using a high-pitched tone of voice and an exaggerated affective facial expression. These manifestations, which are characteristic of dyadic communications (Gergely and Watson, 1996), arise spontaneously in contact with the infant to the extent that the adult is affectively engaged in the relationship and has interiorised an emotional dimension of early development. Another communication resource is the practitioner verbalising the infant's emotional experiences in the first person, as if the infant him/herself were speaking. Stern observed that this modality allows parents to perceive and become more sensitive to the infant's hitherto unnoticed affective states (Stern, 1995). Along the same lines, Dolto (1971) includes the practitioner's verbalisations which are addressed to the infant but intended to be heard by the mother.

Based on the previous, the work presented in the following chapters assumes that, within the setting of a complex transference dynamic which takes place during the paediatric check-up and involves all its protagonists, the way the practitioner establishes eye contact with the infant, listens and talks to it and reacts affectively to his/her initiatives and responses in the interaction conveys the representation to the parents of an infant with a psychic and emotional life. At the same time, this context allows them to integrate new resources in the relationship with the infant, taking the professional's attitude as a reference and as a model of communication, relation and emotional expression.

References

Barba-Müller, E. (2015). *Morphologic brain changes induced by pregnancy: A longitudinal magnetic resonance imaging study* (doctoral thesis). Autonomous University of Barcelona. Doctoral Programme in Psychiatry and Cognitive Neuroscience. https://dialnet.unirioja.es.

Barba-Müller, E., Craddock, S., Carmona, S. and Hoekzema, E. (2018). Brain plasticity in pregnancy and the postpartum period: Links to maternal caregiving and mental health. *Archives of Women's Mental Health, 22*, 289–299.

Benjamin, J. (2002). The rhythm of recognition. *Comments on the Work of Louis Sander. Psychoanalytic Dialogues, 12*(1), 43–53.

Benjamin, J. and Atlas, G. (2014 [2015]). The 'too muchness' of excitement: Sexuality in light of excess, attachment and affect regulation. *The International Journal of Psychoanalysis, 96*(1), 39–63. [+ *IJP Open – Open Peer Review and Debate*, (1), 1–35].

Bleichmar, S. (1995). Entre la producción de subjetividad y la constitución del psiquismo [From parental discourse to symptom specificity in child psychoanalysis]. In A. Sigal (Ed.). *El lugar de los padres en el Psicoanálisis de niños*. Buenos Aires: Lugar, pp. 81–108.

Brazelton, T. (1978). The Brazelton Neonatal behavior assessment scale. *Monographs of the Society for Research in Child Development*, (5–6), 1–13.

Brazelton, T. (1994). Touchpoints: Opportunities for preventing problems in the parent-child relationship. *Acta Paediatrica, 394*(Suppl), 35–39.

Cramer, B. (1990 [1997]). *The scripts parents write and the roles babies play: The importance of being baby (The master work series)/[De profesión bebé]*. New Jersey; London: Jason Aronson; Barcelona: Urano.

Cramer, B. and Palacio Espasa, F. (1993). *La pratique des psychoterapies meres-bébés: Étude clinique et technique [Clinical and technical study]*. Paris: Presses Universitaires de France.

Dolto, F. (1971). *Psychanalise et pédiatrie*. Paris: Editions du Seuil.

Domínguez, M., Cruz, V., Abelleira, M., Amado, A. and Fernández, M. (2009). *Desarrollo evolutivo del neonato: [Developmental development of the neonate]: Clinical utility of the Brazelton Scale. Actas do 10 Congresso Internacional Galego-Português de Psicopedagogia*. Braga: Universidade do Minho.

Emde, R., Gaensbauer, T. and Harmon, R. (1976). Emotional expression in infancy: A bio behavioural study. *Psychological Issues, 10*(1), 1–200.

Fonagy, P., Gergely, G., Jurist, E. and Target, M. (2002). *Affect regulation, mentalization, and the development of the self*. New York: Other Press.

Fox, S., Levitt, P. and Nelson, C. (2010). How the timing and quality of early experiences influence the development of brain architecture. *Child Development, 81*(1), 28–40.

Fraiberg, S., Adelson, E. and Schapito, V. (1975). Ghosts in the nursery: A psychoanalytic approach to the problems of impaired infant-mother relationships. *Journal of the American Academy of Child & Adolescent Psychiatry, 14*(3), 387–421.

Gergely, G. and Watson, J. S. (1996). The social biofeedback theory of parental affect-mirroring: The development of emotional self-awareness and self-control in infancy. *The International Journal of Psychoanalysis, 77*(6), 1181–1212.

Guedeney, A. and Fermanian, J. (2001). A validity and reliability study of assessment and screening for sustained withdrawal reaction in infancy: The alarm distress baby scale. *Infant Mental Health Journal, 22*(5), 559–575.

Harvard University. (2014). *Center on the developing child. A decade of science informing policy: The story of the national scientific council on the developing child*. Cambridge, MA: Harvard University. https://developingchild.harvard.edu/resources/decade-science-informing-policy-story-national-scientific-council-developing-child/ (Accessed 18 December 2020).

Heckman, J. (2015). *Four big benefits of investing in early childhood development*. The Heckman Equation. http://heckmanequation.org/content/resource/4-big-benefits-investing-early-childhood-development.

Keefer, C., Johnson, L. and Minear, S. (2009). Relationship-based practice in the newborn nursery. In J. K. Nugent, B. Petrauskas and T. Brazelton (Eds.). *The infant as a person: Enabling healthy infant development worldwide*. Hoboken: John Wiley & Sons, Inc.

Kreisler, L., Fain, M. and Soulé, M. (1997). *El niño y su cuerpo [The child and its body]: Studies on the psychosomatic clinic of childhood*. Buenos Aires: Amorrortu.

Laplanche, J. (1989). *New foundations for psychoanalysis*. Oxford: Basil Blackwell.

Leblanc, N. and Soulé, M. (1995). La información y capacitación del personal [Staff information and training]. In S. Lebovici and F. Weil Halpern (Eds.). *La psicopatología del lactante [The psychopathology of the infant]*. Buenos Aires: Siglo XXI.

Lebovici, S. (1988a). Fantasmatic interactions and intergenerational transmission. *Infant Mental Health Journal, 9*, 10–19.

Lebovici, S. (1988b). *El Lactante, su madre y el psicoanalista: Las interacciones precoces [The infant, his mother and the psychoanalyst: Early interactions]*. Buenos Aires: Amorrortu.

Lebovici, S. and Weil-Harper, F. (1995). *La psicopatología del bebé [The psychopathology of the baby]*. Buenos Aires: Siglo XXI Ed.

Lewin, K. (1946). Action research and minority problems. *Journal of Social Issues, 2*, 34–46.

Lieberman, A. and Paul, J. (1993). Infant-parent psychotherapy. In C. Zennah (Ed.). *Handbook of infant mental health*. New York; Boston: Guilford, pp. 427–442.

Nugent, J. K. (2015). The newborn behavioural observations (NBO) system as a form of intervention and support for new parents. *Zero to Three Journal, 36*(1), 2–10.

Stern, D. (1985). *The interpersonal world of the infant: A view from psychoanalysis and developmental psychology*. New York: Basic Books.

Stern, D. (1995). *The motherhood constellation: A unified view of parent-infant psychotherapy*. Buenos Aires: Basic Books; Harper Collins.

Tronick, E., Als, H., Adamson, L., Wise, S. and Brazelton, T. (1978). Infant response to entrapment between contradictory messages in face-to-face interaction. *Journal of the American Academy of Child and Adolescent Psychiatry, 17*(1), 1–13.

Winnicott, D. (1941). The observation of infants in a set situation. *International Journal of Psychoanalysis, 22*, 229–249.

Winnicott, D. (1956 [1958]). Chapter XXIV: Primary maternal preoccupation. In *Through paediatrics to psycho-analysis*. New York: Basic Books.

Winnicott, D. (1960). The theory of the parent-infant relationship. *International Journal of Psychoanalysis, 41*, 585–595. [& in *The maturational process and the facilitating environment*. London: Hogarth Press, 1964].

World Health Organization. (2015). *Global strategy for women's, children's and adolescents' health (2016–2030): Survive, thrive, transform*. https://platform.who.int/data/maternal-newborn-child-adolescent-ageing/global-strategy-data#:~:text=This%20Global%20Strategy%20includes%20a,that%20all%20women%2C%20children%2C%20and.

Worthman, C., Tomlinson, M. and Rotheram-Borus, M. (2016). When can parents most influence their child's development? Expert knowledge and perceived local realities. *Social Science & Medicine, 154*, 62–69.

9   Infant withdrawal

A key sign of risk in early emotional development

This chapter takes as its starting point contributions from the observation and investigation of early interactions, in dialogue with psychoanalytic ideas and current scientific knowledge. Against this background, with-drawal behaviour in infants is presented as a key sign of risk in early emo-tional development and child mental health.

Observational studies show that the mother and infant actively seek and sustain interaction through gazes, gestures, vocalisations and facial expres-sions (Emde et al., 1976; Tronick et al., 1978; Brazelton et al., 1975, 1979; Stern, 1985). This scenario is one of preverbal communication, in which both protagonists influence and adapt to each other's approaches and responses, coordinating their experiences and emotions (Tronick, 2007). The rhythm and synchrony of the dyad during this dynamic are expres-sions of shared emotional states or, in Winnicott's (1967) terms, of "living and feeling together" or an "experience of mutuality" between mother and infant. These early experiences are essential elements for organisation of the incipient psyche and the process of subjectivation (Stern, 1985). Fur-thermore, current researchers emphasise that the synchrony of the dyad during the first year of life provides the infant with a critical social experi-ence for the development of empathy and the social capacity that under-lies human relationships throughout life (Feldman, 2007). In addition, the infant's social capacity and interest in exploring the world relate to the experience of shared emotional states in the synchronous exchanges of the dyad (Emde, 1998).

On the other hand, repeated and lasting difficulties in synchrony dis-tress the infant, causing an avoidance reaction towards the relationship, which implies an inhibition of social capacity, in other words withdrawal behaviour (Guedeney, 1997, 2000, 2007). This situation always constitutes a risk for a child's development and mental health. According to studies by Soulé et al. (1995), difficulties in early relationships result in a loss of opportunities for development, which sets in and persists early, when the child is not quite 1 year old. Moreover, a Uruguayan study with a sample of more than a thousand children under the age of 2 (Interdisciplinary Group of Psychosocial Studies, 1996) identifies inhibition in social interaction as

DOI: 10.4324/9781032614823-12

one of the early indicators of delays in child development. In accordance with these contributions, science currently associates adverse conditions in the early relationship with a state of "toxic stress" in the infant, which produces damage at a neurobiological level and lasting difficulties in learning, behaviour, and physical and mental health (National Scientific Council on the Developing Child, Harvard University, 2014).

Based on this knowledge, the work presented in the following chapters assumes that inhibition of social capacity or withdrawal behaviour on the part of the infant is a sign of early emotional distress associated with difficulties in the dyadic relationship and constitute an alarm signal for mental health and development as a whole. From this perspective, early detection of the first signs of infant withdrawal is thus a key element for carrying out timely interventions and a preventive approach with the infant and its parents, with the participation and commitment of primary care professionals.

Withdrawn behaviour in infants, early psychopathology and development

Historically, various psychoanalytic authors have identified withdrawn behaviour in infants to be a clinical element of early psychopathology. The study of this subject from various perspectives and the analysis of its theoretical implications are of relevance in relation to the origins of psychic life and childhood psychopathology. However, these issues go beyond the purpose of this communication, in which I merely intend to make some brief references which I find particularly significant for the work presented next.

Moreover, Spitz (1945) includes withdrawal behaviour as a central aspect of anaclitic depression, thus defining a clinical condition that occurs in the infant as a consequence of emotional deprivation due to a sudden and prolonged separation from its mother. This author observes that after two months of such a separation, the infant shows rejection of contact, rigidity in facial expression and motor delay, and that these symptoms become accentuated over time if the separation situation persists. He also points out that this disorder reverts quickly if the child is reunited with a maternal figure before a critical period, which he places as within a few months.

In contrast, Fraiberg (1982) describes the infant's withdrawal behaviour within a range of early pathological defences that manifest when confronted with a maternal presence that is perceived as threatening and distressing. This scenario includes extreme situations of neglect and abuse by parental figures with severe psychopathology. Fraiberg observes that these infants never or rarely seek eye contact with their mother, do not respond with a smile to her face or voice, nor do they vocalise when addressing her, as would be expected in a healthy infant. He adds that they do not seek the physical proximity of the mother even when they are able to crawl or walk, and that in times of need or distress they do not turn to the mother for relief and consolation. These observations lead Fraiberg to suggest that where one would expect the infant to seek a mother figure and a relationship, instead avoidance occurred. For this author, the avoidance of the relationship is based on the infant's experience and implies a tendency towards the expectation and anticipation of danger because the mother figure is associated with a threat to the child's functioning.

In another context, Benjamin and Atlas (2015) also mention withdrawal behaviour as a primary defence, referring to a disconnection or flight from the relationship in the infant exposed to disconcerting and overwhelming maternal responses. Finally, returning to traditional Freudian terms, Salomonsson (2016) studies gaze avoidance as a defence mechanism for infants confronted with a frightening relationship. From another perspective, withdrawal behaviour is considered to be a decrease in attachment which becomes gradually generalised and is expressed as low reactivity towards the environment (Zeanah et al., 2000).

On the other hand, in the field of dyadic observation, the *still-face* video-filmed experimental situation proposed by Tronick et al. (1978) paradigmatically shows the initiatives and resources of the infant in the interaction (Brazelton et al., 1974, 1979), while also allowing us to assess his extreme sensitivity and dependence on maternal responses. Confronted with the mother's lack of facial expressiveness, his range of resources is rapidly reduced. Although the infant's initial reactions are active and the child shows signs of protest, such as crying, screaming and gestures to attract the adult's attention, observations show that if the maternal figure continues to fail to respond, the infant becomes disorganised, looks away and disengages from the relationship (Tronick et al., 1978). Later studies identify this reaction to any unexpected and unpredictable maternal response, which by omission or overstimulation alters the infant's rhythm and expectation in the interaction (Murray et al., 1993; Murray and Cooper, 1997). In the habitual and daily dynamics of the dyad, synchrony coexists and alternates with these failures in communication, in the face of which the mother and the infant spontaneously take actions that restore the rhythm of the relationship (Tronick et al., 1978). However, when the alterations in rhythm and synchrony are repeated and become long-lasting, and the resources of the dyad are not sufficient to generate new encounters, then withdrawal behaviour progressively sets in for the infant, compromising his or her social capacity, which becomes inhibited to an extreme extent (Guedeney, 2007).

As Fraiberg (1982) points out, although relationship avoidance protects the infant from a distressing relational experience, it also exposes him or her to experiences of isolation, helplessness, and distress. At a time when the maternal figure constitutes an essential element for the incipient psyche, the infant is left alone and, therefore, without resources to cope with his urgent needs (Fraiberg, 1982), the intensity of his impulses (Fonagy, 2002) and the uncertainty of external stimuli (Emde, 1998). This situation always implies emotional distress and has consequences for early psychological functioning.

Longitudinal research in recent years reveals the consequences of infant withdrawal behaviour in the development of their abilities and mental health. A study carried out in Australia found that a group of infants presenting with withdrawal behaviour at six months old had social and cognitive problems and difficulties in language acquisition at 3 years old (Milne et al., 2009). Research carried out in France also showed that withdrawal behaviour in 1-year-old infants led to difficulties in emotional regulation and behavioural disorders at 5 years old (Guedeney et al., 2014), as well as language delays (Guedeney et al., 2016). Moreover, if early detection and intervention do not take place, infant withdrawal behaviour can become a precursor to childhood depression, or even usher in the major psychopathological diagnostic categories of early childhood, such as autism spectrum disorders, anxiety disorders and developmental delays (Guedeney and Vermillard, 2004).

Other recent studies identify risk groups of infants who present greater withdrawal behaviour due to multiple factors that affect early relationships. For example, various types of organic difficulties in the newborn emotionally impact the parents and interfere with the relationship (Re et al., 2010). The same occurs in the case of premature babies, whose very biological condition complicates the modality, times and rhythms of interaction. In relation to parental figures and taken to the extreme of psychopathology, different studies show that the infant is more withdrawn in situations in which the mother is depressed (Matthey et al., 2005; Braarud et al., 2013) and where both parents are experiencing mental health difficulties (Mäntymaa et al., 2008).

Finally, a relevant issue for the work presented in the following chapters refers to the psychosocial risk conditions that affect the early relationship. Studies carried out in different regions show that infants from these groups present greater withdrawal behaviour than other populations, due to the negative impact of contextual conditions on family dynamics and the parent-infant bond (Guedeney et al., 2013). These data confirm that conditions of psychosocial vulnerability lead to a greater risk for the development of infant capacities and child mental health from a very early age, thus accentuating the inequality of opportunities from the outset (Lebovici and Weil-Harper, 1995; Sameroff et al., 1999).

Taking this reality into account, caring for early relations in contexts of psychosocial risk becomes especially relevant for the infant and its future possibilities. Current studies show that infants who are a few months old and have a history of responsive and sensitive relationships have more resources to cope with adversity than younger infants, who more quickly become disorganised and disengaged (Feldman, 2007). These observations have led researchers to recognise a certain protective effect that early relational experiences acquire for the infant. Along the same lines, research from the Center on the Developing Child at Harvard University (2014) reaffirms the importance of the quality of early relational experiences, concluding that "providing stable, responsive and supportive relationships during the first years of life can prevent or even reverse the detrimental effects of adversity in situations of psychosocial vulnerability, with lasting benefits for learning, behaviour and health".

Clinical manifestations and difficulties in the early detection of infant withdrawal

According to studies in early development, the healthy infant shows interest and curiosity in the people around him and solicits attention and responses through looks, smiles, gestures and vocalisations. In contrast, when an infant is withdrawn, this availability for the relationship is affected, and there is a decrease in expressiveness and communicative capacity, which can become inhibited (Guedeney, 2007). The latter state creates a clinical picture of a distant infant who is aloof from her surroundings and inaccessible to contact. These extreme conditions which imply a greater risk for infant development and mental health do not occur suddenly. However, the progressive establishment of withdrawal behaviour in the infant's relational modality makes its first expressions hard to detect, so it may go unnoticed in the clinical setting, until withdrawal becomes more marked and invasive. Taking this aspect into account, an observational tool has been created for early detection of such phenomena. The *Alarme Détresse Bébé* scale (ADBB, Guedeney and Fermanian, 2001) is a key tool in the work presented next.

In an initial stage of exploring the use of this tool in Uruguay, a study was carried out with a population at high psychosocial risk, from the metropolitan area of the country's capital. The methodological advisors for this work were R. Emde and P. Fonagy, who were mentors of the project in the IPA Research Training Programme, which took place in London, in 2009 (Bonifacino et al., 2014). The results obtained showed that in the traditional well child visit, the infant's withdrawal behaviour was only detected if it was evident and severe, with a major inhibition of social ability. However, the first signs of this went unnoticed under clinical observation, so timely intervention could not take place. This study also revealed that when there are no resources available for early detection and intervention, and the infant continues to be exposed to distressing situations, withdrawal behaviour does not reverse of its own accord. On the contrary, it tends to increase. Accordingly, of 37 infants evaluated, 40% showed signs of withdrawal behaviour between the ages of 2 and 6 months, which is an alarming picture. However, even more worryingly, in a second evaluation of this same group carried out two months later on infants between 4 and 8 months old, withdrawal behaviour had increased to 57%.

Moreover, all these infants attended regular well-baby visits and were in good shape in terms of physical growth and development, so it was reasonable to suppose that the withdrawal detected was rooted in relational and emotional issues. These data lead us to propose that, although current paediatrics recognises developmental care as an important objective and guidelines are created for its assessment during the well-baby visit, the infant's relational abilities are not usually considered significant elements of this. As a consequence, this is a lost opportunity for preventive intervention to reduce risk in early emotional development and child mental health. Another important fact that emerges from this study is that training paediatricians in the importance of early interactions for development and the ADBB scale provides greater tools to carry out early detections and timely interventions arising from the well-baby visit, leading to an increase in the quality of care (Bonifacino et al., 2014).

From my experience as a psychoanalyst who works with young children with severe disorders, I understand that it is relevant for the care of infant mental health that professionals who are on the first level of care have resources for the early detection of signs of infant's emotional suffering and of his/her difficulties in relationships with the other. Only thus can timely interventions be carried out at the necessary levels of care, avoiding greater suffering for the child and her family. If these conditions are not met, however, the outcome of the infant's withdrawal behaviour may be severe psychopathology of early childhood, as was the case with the young children to whom I refer in the first section of this book. In most of these situations, the difficulties were only detected between the ages of two and three, after the children had started pre-school. The child's lack of relational resources and functional delays became evident in the challenges of an educational setting, in which the child is required to integrate into a social framework and take part in recreational activities. As current basic principles of neuroscience point out, early preventive intervention is more efficient and has more favourable outcomes than rehabilitation carried out later in life (Center on the Developing Child at Harvard University, 2014). This knowledge poses the challenge of expanding the resources of professionals of the first level of care for the benefit of a culture of detection of risk and promotion of the early relationship, which reaches the different scenarios of care for the infant and their parents, from the newborn well-baby visit.

Early detection of infant withdrawal behaviour: the Alarm Détresse Bébé scale

The ADBB scale is an infant observation guide for detecting withdrawal behaviour from its first clinical expression. This tool was created in France in 2001 by Antoine Guedeney, who is a professor emeritus, MD. PhD professor of child and adolescent psychiatry and perinatality and PhD in child development. This author has training and professional experience as a paediatrician, child psychiatrist and psychoanalyst and has been in charge of child psychopathology units in public services caring for infants and their families. In my view, this tool is a product of his theoretical background and clinical practice in all these fields, combined with an in-depth study of infant withdrawal behaviour. From an observational record, and therefore shareable with other disciplines, the ADBB scale enables information to be obtained on a key element for children's mental health, such as the relational availability of the infant. This condition allows an insight into the dynamics of the early relationship, at the same time forming the basis of the early intersubjective processes inherent to the origins of psychic life, emotional development and the process of subjectivation.

This tool proposes the observation of eight aspects or items related to the social capacity of the infant in the relationship with the professional (Guedeney and Fermanian, 2001). These components include an assessment of facial expressiveness, the infant's initiatives to seek and sustain eye contact, the naturalness and flexibility of her movements, and her ability to express herself with vocalisations. All these are categorised on a continuum which favourably assesses the infant's spontaneous display of such expressions, while at the opposite extreme it considers her inhibition and lack of response to the professional's initiatives. Complementing these aspects, the tool also positively evaluates the quality of the infant's response in terms of the liveliness and immediacy of his reactions to stimuli. In contrast, if the infant displays automatic and stereotypical movements that isolate him from the relationship, these acquire a negative connotation in reference to Spitz's observations in infants with affective deprivation (1945).

Finally, in my opinion the last two items to be evaluated give the tool a clinical profile that enriches it and distinguishes it from purely mechanical observation. These items indirectly involve the professional in the scene actively and with their own emotional aspects as an instrument to discover the infant's resources in the relationship. The first of these evaluates the infant's capacity to engage in the relationship with the professional, which in turn requires the availability and sensitivity of the professional to enable such an encounter. The second, in contrast, evaluates the infant's ability to deploy initiatives that arouse interest and attract attention and that generate pleasant feelings in the professional. These components of the scale promote in the clinician a movement of self-observation which allows him to be aware of his own emotional experiences in the relationship with the infant, thus placing the vicissitudes of the doctor-patient relationship centre stage during the well-child visit. The implications of these circumstances in clinical practice are relevant in the work presented next.

ADBB is a simple and accessible tool after a brief training period. It was created to be used in common situations for the infant and its parents, such as the well-baby visit. This context offers a limited observation time, which proves to be a positive aspect in this case and accords with Lebovici's (Lebovici and Weil-Harper, 1995) recommendation to observe the infant for short periods, accommodating the rapid variation in his or her level of attention. Furthermore, the universal sequence of clinical procedures of the well-baby visit allows infants of the same age to be compared with each other, or the same infant over time. These two resources have been used in the work presented in the following chapters.

The ADBB scale was originally presented as a screening instrument to identify infants at risk in their emotional development, with the suggestion to investigate the causes and guide a referral (Guedeney and Fermanian, 2001; Guedeney and Vermillard, 2004). In agreement with this perspective, Ozonoff et al. (2010) suggest incorporating measures of the infant's social repertoire into the periodic developmental evaluation so that risk cases can be identified.

However, work in training professionals from public health centres carried out in Uruguay since 2006 expands the use of this tool, recognising its usefulness not only for screening purposes but also to promote a more comprehensive concept of health check, which includes infant mental health care and early emotional development promotion, starting with the newborn well-baby visits (Bonifacino et al., 2011, 2014, 2023).

References

Benjamin, J. and Atlas, G. (2014). The 'too muchness' of excitement: Sexuality in light of excess, attachment and affect regulation. *IJP Open – Open Peer Review and Debate, 1*, 1–35. [+ *The International Journal of Psychoanalysis*, (1), 39–63, 2015].

Bonifacino, N., Lezama, G., Nauar, M., Llaguno, N. and Simó, S. (2023). Detección precoz de desviaciones y promoción de las habilidades sociales el lactante con la escala ADBB durante el seguimiento pediátrico. Experiencia en un centro de salud pública de alta vulnerabilidad social. Experiencia en un centro de salud pública de alta vulnerabilidad social [Early detection of deviations and promotion of social skills in infants with the ADBB scale during the paediatric follow-up. Experience in a health centre with high social vulnerability]. *Archivos Pediatría de Uruguay, 94*(2), e218. https://doi.org/10.31134/AP.94.2.

Bonifacino, N., Musetti, D., Plevak, A. and Schelotto, M. (2011). La consultation en pédiatrie: la première approche à la santé mentale des enfants. *Devenir, 23*(2), 117–127. https://doi.org/10.3917/dev.112.0117.

Bonifacino, N., Plevak, A., Musetti, D. and Silveira, A. (2014). Retraimiento sostenido: Un indicador de riesgo en el desarrollo temprano [Sustained withdrawal behaviour: An indicator of risk in early development]. Detección e intervención en el primer nivel con la escala ADBB [Detection and intervention at the first level with the ADBB scale]. Experiencia en dos centros de salud pública del área metropolitana [Experience in two public health centres in the metropolitan area]. *Archivos Pediatría de Uruguay, 85*(1), 30–38.

Braarud, H., Slinning, K., Moe, V., Smith, L., Vanned, U., Guedeney, A. and Heimann, M. (2013). Relationship between social withdrawal symptoms in full-term and premature infants and depressive symptoms in mother: A longitudinal study. *Infant Mental Health Journal, 34*(6), 532–541.

Brazelton, T., Koslowski, B. and Main, M. (1974). Origins of reciprocity. In M. Lewis and L. Rosenblum (Eds.). *Mother infant interaction*. New York: Wiley, pp. 57–70.

Brazelton, T., Tronick, E., Adamson, L., Als, H. and Wise, S. (1975). Early mother-infant reciprocity. In *Ciba foundation symposium: Parent-infant interaction* (Vol. 33). Amsterdam: Elsevier, pp. 137–154.

Brazelton, T., Yogman, M., Als, H. and Tronick, E. (1979). Joint regulation of neonate-parent behaviour. In E. Tronick (Ed.). *Social interchange in infancy*. Baltimore: University Park Press, pp. 7–22.

Center on the Developing Child at Harvard University. (2014). *A decade of science informing policy: The story of the national scientific council on the developing child*. http://www.developingchild.net.

Emde, R. (1998). Yendo hacia adelante: Las influencias integradoras de los procesos afectivos en el desarrollo y en el psicoanálisis [Going forward: The integrative influences of affective processes in development and psychoanalysis]. *Psicoanálisis APdeBA, 20*(3), 473–516.

Emde, R., Gaensbauer, T. and Harmon, R. (1976). Emotional expression in infancy: A biobehavioral study. *Psychological Issues, 10*(1), 1–200.

Feldman, R. (2007). Parent-infant synchrony and the construction of shared timing; physiological precursors, developmental outcomes, and risk conditions. *Journal of Child Psychology and Psychiatry, 48*(3–4), 329–354.

Fonagy, P. (2002). *Affect regulation, mentalisation and the development of the self*. New York: Other Press.

Fraiberg, S. (1982). Pathological defences in infancy. *Psychoanalytical Quarterly, 51*, 612–635.

Guedeney, A. (1997). From early withdrawal behaviour reaction to infant depression: A baby alone does exist. *Infant Mental Health Journal, 18*(4), 339–349.

Guedeney, A. (2000). Infant depression and withdrawal: Clinical assessment. In J. D. Osofsky and H. E. Fitzgerald (Eds.). *WAIMH handbook of infant mental health* (Vol. 4). New York: Wiley, pp. 455–484.

Guedeney, A. (2007). Withdrawal behaviour and depression in infancy. *Infant Mental Health Journal, 28*(4), 393–408.

Guedeney, A. and Fermanian, J. (2001). A validity and reliability study of assessment and screening for sustained withdrawal reaction in infancy. The alarm distress baby scale (ADBB). *Infant Mental Health Journal, 22*(5), 559–575.

Guedeney, A., Forhan, A., Larroque, B., Agostini de, M., Pingault, J.-B., Heude, B., et al. (2016). Social withdrawal behaviour at one year of age is associated with delays in reaching language milestones in the Eden mother-child cohort study. *PLoS One, 11*(7).

Guedeney, A., Matthey, S. and Puura, K. (2013). Social withdrawal behaviour in infancy: A history of the concept and a review of published studies using the alarm distress baby scale. *Infant Mental Health Journal, 34*(6), 516–531. https://doi.org/10.1002/imhj.21412.

Guedeney, A., Pingault, J. B., Thorr, A., Larroque, B. and EDEN Mother-Child Cohort Study Group. (2014). Social withdrawal at one year is associated with emotional and behavioural problems at 3 and 5 years: The Eden mother-child cohort study. *European Child & Adolescent Psychiatry, 12*, 1181–1188.

Guedeney, A. and Vermillard, M. (2004). L'echelle ADBB; intérêt en recherché et en clinique de l'evaluation du comportement de portrait relationnel du jeune enfant. *Médicine Enfance, 20*(11), 364–371.

Interdisciplinary Group of Psychosocial Studies. (1996). *Cuidando el potencial el futuro: El desarrollo de niños preescolares en familias pobres en Uruguay [Caring for the future's potential: Preschool children's development in poor families in Uruguay]* (L. Schwartzmann, Ed.). Montevideo: University of the Republic.

Lebovici, S. and Weil-Halpern, F. (1995). *La psicopatología del bebé [The psychopathology of the baby]*. Buenos Aires: Siglo XXI Ed.

Mäntymaa, M., Puura, K., Luomai, I., Kaukonnen, P., Salmelin, R. and Tamminent, T. (2008). Infant's social withdrawal behaviour and parent's mental health. *Infant Behavior and Development, 31*, 606–613.

Matthey, S., Guedeney, A., Starakis, N. and Barnett, B. (2005). Assessing the social behaviour of infants: Use of the ADBB scale and relationship to mother's mood. *Infant Mental Health Journal, 26*, 442–458.

Milne, L., Greenway, P., Guedeney, A. and Larroque, B. (2009). Long term developmental impact of social withdrawal in infants. *Infant Behavior and Development,* 32(2), 159–166.

Murray, L. and Cooper, P. (1997). *Postpartum depression and child development.* New York: The Guilford.

Murray, L., Kempton, C., Woolgar, M. and Hooper, R. (1993). Depressed mothers' speech to their infants and its relationship to infant gender and cognitive development. *Journal of Child Psychology and Psychiatry, 34*, 1083–1101.

National Scientific Council on the Developing Child. (2014). *Excessive stress disrupts the architecture of the developing brain: Working paper 3.* Cambridge, MA: Harvard University. https://developingchild.harvard.edu/resources/wp3/ (Accessed 18 December 2020).

Ozonoff, S., Iosif, A., Baguio, F., Cook, I., Moore Hill, M., Hutman, T., Rogers, S., Rozga, A., Sangha, S., Marian, M., Steinfeld, M. and Young, G. (2010). A prospective study of the emergence of early behavioral signs of autism. *Journal of the American Academy of Child & Adolescent Psychiatry, 49*(3), 256–266.

Re, J., Dean, S., Menahem, S. and Paul, C. (2010). Holding mothers in mind mothers holding babies in mind through medical and surgical treatment for children. *Infant Mental Health Journal, 31*(3), 104.

Salomonsson, B. (2016, February). Infantile defences in parent-infant psychotherapy: The example of gaze avoidance. *The International Journal of Psychoanalysis, 97*(1), 65–88. https://doi.org/10.1111/1745-8315.12331; Epub: 19 May 2015; PMID: 25988970.

Sameroff, A., Bartko, W., Baldwin, A., Baldwin, C. and Seifer, R. (1999). Family and social influences on the development of child competence. In M.Lewis and C.Feiring (Eds.). *Families, risk, and competence.* Mahwah, NJ: Lawrence Erlbaum Associates, pp. 161–186.

Soulé, M., Noel, J. and Frichet, A. (1995). Le travail préventif auprès de la de la famille en faveur du très jeune enfant. In S.Lebovici and F.Weil-Halpern (Eds.). *Psychopathologie du bébé.* Buenos Aires: Siglo XXI.

Spitz, R. (1945). Hospitalism: An inquiry into the genesis of psychiatric conditions in early childhood. *Psychoanalytic Study of the Child, 1*, 53–74.

Stern, D. (1985). *The interactional world of the infant: A view from psychoanalysis and developmental psychology.* New York: Basic Books.

Tronick, E. (2007). *Interactive mismatch and repair: Challenges to the coping infant. In The neurobehavioral and social-emotional development of infants and children.* New York, NY: Norton & Company.

Tronick, E., Als, H., Adamson, L., Wise, S. and Brazelton, T. (1978). Infant response to entrapment between contradictory messages in face-to-face interaction. *Journal of the American Academy of Child and Adolescent Psychiatry, 17*(1), 1–13.

Winnicott, D. (1967 [1971]). Mirror role of mother and family in child development. In D. Winnicott (Ed.). *Playing and reality.* London: Tavistock Publications.

Zeanah, C., Boris, N., Bakshi, S. and Lieberman, A. (2000). *Disorders of attachment.* New York: Wiley.

10 Training of the health team for a preventive approach to children's mental health

This chapter describes a training programme that expands the resources of first care level professionals who take care of infants and parents to facilitate early detection of risk and promote early emotional development, while fostering interdisciplinary dialogue based on observation and detection of infant withdrawal.

This programme was started in 2006 at public health centres in areas of high psychosocial risk in the metropolitan zone of Montevideo, Uruguay, having received research grants from the International Psychoanalytic Association in 2010 and 2012. In these phases, paediatricians from two primary care centres were trained, and the impact of the application of the practitioners' new knowledge during the well-baby visit was evaluated to assess its benefit for infant well-being (Bonifacino et al., 2011, 2014). In a later study, conducted in another public health centre which offered paediatric care, this training was also extended to practitioners from different disciplines working with infants and their parents (Bonifacino et al., 2023). On all these occasions, the training was carried out by the author, sometimes accompanied by other practitioners.

Moreover, this training also took place at the Paediatrics Society of Uruguay, with accreditation from the Graduate School of the Faculty of Medicine of the University of the Republic (2012–2015), and was selected by the Competitive Funds of the Uruguayan Medical Union for its Continuing Professional Development department in its two editions in 2021 and 2022. These placements in renowned local medical institutions enabled this training to be given to a large number of paediatricians, family doctors, neuro-paediatricians and other medical practitioners in Uruguay. In some of these training courses, paediatricians and a family doctor who had participated in previous courses and had experience carrying them out in paediatric well-baby visits were integrated into the teaching team. In addition, this training was included in university master's studies in clinical child psychology and educational psychology at the Catholic University of Uruguay (from 2012–2018) and at the Faculty of Psychology of the University of the Republic (in 2014) respectively. Finally, training took place through various professional associations for psychologists, psychomotor

DOI: 10.4324/9781032614823-13

therapists, speech therapists, social workers, early childhood educators and teachers, as well as medical practitioners and students from different disciplines in contact with infants and young children, both in Uruguay and abroad.

This initiative arises from an interest in promoting an interdisciplinary dialogue between psychoanalysis and practitioners who are on the front line of infant and young child care. This setting includes health services and educational or day-care centres, where infants and young children often spend many hours daily, which generally coincide with their parents' working hours. In fact, my initial contact with the ADBB scale (Chapter 9) was based on certain concerns and worries that arose from my role as the person responsible for the mental health of a large number of infants and young children who attended an institution with this profile. This institution received more than a hundred children from the ages of 2 to 24 months, who spent up to eight or nine hours a day in the care of a large team of educators and early childhood educators (Bonifacino, 2010). Although the practitioners' commitment was beyond reproach, in my view this collective care framework interfered with the individual attention required by each infant, potentially jeopardising their healthy emotional development. In this context, questions arose for me: what resources could I provide to frontline educators so that they would be able to detect signs of emotional distress or suffering in the infant? Or on what shared basis could a dialogue be established with the paediatrician and the child nutritionist who shared institutional responsibility for the health and proper development of the infant who attended this institution? The answer to these questions came in the form of the ADBB scale, which advocates, through infant observation, for the early detection of signs of infant withdrawal behaviour.

I was first trained in the use of this tool in 2005 by Dr Guedeney, at the invitation of Dr Mónica Oliver, an esteemed colleague from the Argentine Psychoanalytic Association, who is unfortunately no longer with us. At that time, she was head of the Department of Psychopathology at the German Hospital in Buenos Aires, where she organised the training for her team members. Since then, we have both been endorsed by Dr Guedeney to train other practitioners in the use of the tool. The training programme presented in this chapter is my personal line of work with the ADBB scale. This line proposes a training model in this tool for its incorporation into the first care level, with the aim of early detection of withdrawal and the promotion of early emotional development from the paediatric well-baby visit for newborn infants. To this end, training on the ADBB scale is complemented by an interdisciplinary perspective on the importance of interactions for infant development and mental health and strategies to promote infant social skills during paediatric well-baby visits. This proposal is in line with the recommendations and guidelines of the American Academy of Paediatrics (AAP) (2019) and the World Association for Infant Mental Health (WAIMH) (Puura et al., 2018), in reference to providing resources to paediatricians and other first-level health practitioners for a preventive approach to infant mental health.

I shall describe this training programme in the context of a larger study, carried out in a public health care centre in Uruguay, which gave us an insight into the experience of practitioners from different disciplines in carrying out training and integrating it into clinical practice. This study also assessed the effect of this approach in the paediatric follow-up of a group of infants. This issue will be addressed in the next chapter.

Professional training programme for detection of withdrawal and the promotion of early emotional development with the ADBB scale in a public health centre of high social vulnerability

Public health and education services are available in Uruguay, and all newborns have access to regular well-baby visits, which are carried out by paediatricians or family doctors, with or without nursing staff present. The Misurraco Health Centre is located in a highly socially vulnerable area on the outskirts of Montevideo (Marconi neighborhood), with a high degree of child poverty. At least 40% of the population has unmet basic needs, and figures from 2016 show that 47.4% of children aged 0–4 live below the poverty line. This area has had the highest rate of endemic violence in the country for at least ten years. These circumstances lead to high staff turnover at the care centre. The directors invited all practitioners working with infants to the training course, and 22 of the 25 who did so participated. This group included five paediatricians, seven general practitioners, two paediatric nutritionists, four paediatric nurses, a paediatric dentist, a child psychiatrist, a psychologist and a social worker.

The training was conducted over three five-hour meetings weekly, and subsequent fortnightly two-hour workshops for six months. These activities were carried out within the care unit and during the practitioners' working hours. During the first meeting, the instructor presented video footage of a well-baby visit and asked the practitioners to make individual observations to identify whether or not the infant presented a developmental risk, recording the factors which led to their assessment. This same infant would be observed again by the practitioners at the end of the ADBB training, this time using the knowledge acquired.

Table 10.1 describes the components of the training programme and the associated workshops.

Component 1. The impact of early interactions on infant development and mental health. This theme was presented from interdisciplinary perspective, with current contributions from neuroscience (Shonkoff et al., 2021; Boyce et al., 2021; Worthman et al., 2010; Fox et al., 2010) and psychoanalytic insights into early emotional development (Winnicott, 1956, 1960; Fonagy et al., 2002) and the parent-infant relationship (Stern, 1995).

Table 10.1 Components and contents of the training programme.

Components	Contents
Impact of early interactions on development and mental health. 1st meeting.	*Parent-infant interactions, infant development and mental health.* • Infant social skills and relationship dependence. • Enduring difficulties in the synchrony of the mother-infant dyad: consequences for development and mental health. • Infant withdrawal: a sign of risk in early emotional development. Clinical presentation, causes and consequences. *Material: presentation and video material provided by the teacher.*
The ADBB scale. 2nd and 3rd meetings.	*ADBB training* • Presentation of characteristics and conditions for using the ADBB. • Practice in assessing 25 infants aged 2 to 24 months with varying degrees of withdrawal: Module 1. Group assessment of 6-month-old infants with guidance from the teacher. Module 2 to Module 4: Individual assessment of infants by age range, with subsequent group discussion (12–24 months, 6–12 months, and 2–5 months). Module 5: Assessment of the knowledge acquired to apply the ADBB. *Material: manual, instructions and coding sheets to apply the ADBB scale. Video footage provided by the teacher.*
Integration of training into clinical practice and strategies to promote infant social skills during the paediatric visit. Fortnightly meetings for six months.	*Supervised application of the ADBB scale to infants during the paediatric well-baby visit.* A guide to strategies for facilitating communication with the infant during paediatric assessment: • Paying direct attention to the infant by seeking eye contact, talking to the infant and asking questions in the form of a dialogue. • Sustaining a committed relationship with the infant taking into account his or her reactions and initiatives. • Describing aloud and making sense of the infant's gestures, movements, facial expressions and/or vocalisations in the interaction with the practitioner. • Identifying and naming the emotions that the infant expresses throughout the review (*"I think you don't like this . . . you are angry", "You like to be talked to . . . and you like to talk!"*) • The practitioner reflects the infant's emotions throughout the assessment with their tone of voice and facial expressions, giving sensitive responses. • Showing parents the infant's interest and pleasure in the relationship. • Pointing out the infant's gestures, movements and/or glances aimed at seeking contact with the mother/father (*"You are looking at Mummy . . .", "You want to go to Mummy . . ."*). *Material: Footage of infants undergoing paediatric well-baby visit with participating practitioners.*

In this context, video footage of the "still face" experience (Tronick, 1978) and some footage from Spitz's (1945) research with institutionalised infants were presented for observation and to generate dialogue among the participants. In general, this video footage has an impact on medical practitioners, enabling them to identify the extreme sensitivity and dependency of the infant in the relationship, as well as the emotional dimension of early development. As Leblanc and Soulé (1995) state, this emotional dimension incorporated by the doctor carrying out the well-baby visit is an indispensable condition for any preventive action in infant mental health.

Component 2. Training in the ADBB scale for the early detection of child withdrawal. The ADBB training model described in the next section incorporates suggestions from Dr Guedeney (personal communication, Buenos Aires, 2005) and is conducted in a group setting. It consists of the presentation of the characteristics of the tool and some general guidelines to facilitate its use, followed by the observation and evaluation with ADBB of 25 infants aged 2 to 24 months, with different degrees of withdrawal. This video footage includes no more than ten minutes of the doctor-infant interaction during the well-baby visit, when the practitioner performs a routine medical examination with the mother or father present.

The infants were presented in five modules with five videos each. The first module presented five infants who were the same age (6 months), ranging from a healthy display of interaction skills to the extreme situation of severe and invasive withdrawal, with high developmental risk. These infants were assessed using the ADBB in a group setting, under the teacher's guidance. From the second module onwards, the infants were presented in decreasing age ranges, taking into account the greater difficulty of detecting signs of withdrawal in younger infants. Each practitioner made his or her own assessment of each infant using the ADBB, subsequently opening up discussion of the items of the scale among all participants. In accordance with Lebovici's (Lebovici and Weil-Harper, 1995) experience, during this training, observation of the infant by physical and mental health practitioners allowed the physician's attention to be directed towards aspects which tend to go unnoticed, or to be taken for granted in the clinical situation. However, while this training aims to provide practitioners with resources to identify infant behaviours that constitute warning signs, it is also equally important to differentiate these behavioural signs from others that can be attributed to temperamental factors and which if not recognised as such, as Carey (2010) warns, can lead to a mistaken early overdiagnosis, resulting in suffering and harm to the child and his or her family.

The final module of this training on the ADBB scale evaluates the skills acquired by the practitioners in the use of the tool. For this purpose, five infants between 2 and 24 months of age with different degrees of withdrawal are presented by the trainer in a randomised manner to be assessed by the practitioners with ADBB scale. This material includes the 6-month-old infant who had been assessed by the practitioners prior to the training. At that time, 8 of the 22 participating practitioners considered the infant to be developmentally at risk, while after the training all identified the infant as developmentally at risk by detecting signs of withdrawal. As is often the case in these training sessions, the practitioners achieved 80% reliability in the use of the tool, which is a prerequisite for clinical use.

At the end of the ADBB training, major episodes of social violence in the neighbourhood put the continuity of the care centre and the integrity of its staff at risk. This situation caused most of the operative staff at the institution to abandon their posts. Thus, the final phase of the training was concentrated on the practitioners who were still working at the health centre.

Component 3. Integration of training into clinical practice and strategies to promote infant emotional development. Four paediatricians, a family doctor, a child nutritionist and a paediatric nurse participated in bi-weekly meetings with the teacher for six months, strengthening their skills in the use of the ADBB scale with supervised practice and incorporating resources to promote the infant's social skills during the well-baby visit.

During this phase, 76 infants between the ages of 2 and 5 months were filmed during their well-baby visit with the team's paediatricians and family doctor. The video footage was used in the bi-weekly meetings, in which each professional assessed each infant according to the ADBB scale, identifying cases of withdrawal. The teacher also presented a strategy guide that facilitated the doctor's communication with the infant during the clinical check-up, based on a sensitive and lively interaction. These strategies involved the practitioner's active approach in seeking contact with the infant, stimulating his or her reactions and encouraging a display of emotions and social skills. The practitioners were encouraged to establish interaction with each infant in a personalised way, based on the contents of the training.

The use of these strategies was also indirectly aimed at the parents present in the clinical situation (Brazelton, 1994), making use of the doctor-patient communication to present a relationship model that recognised and responded to the infant's emotional experiences (Chapter 8).

This approach is in line with recent proposals in paediatrics to focus paediatric care on safe, stable and nurturing relationships to buffer the effects of adversity on infant development (Garner and Yogman, 2021). In the same vein, current perspectives on physical and mental health (Shah et al., 2011) highlight the importance of a relational approach in primary paediatric care to optimise early socio-emotional development. In this context, the practitioner's sensitivity in interacting with the infant during routine well-baby visits is described as an essential element in facilitating emotional bonding between the infant and parent (Keefer et al., 2009).

Practitioners implemented these strategies for six months during routine monthly well-baby visits, and videos were subsequently taken of the infants again when they were between 8 and 11 months old. During this period, it was left to the discretion of each practitioner to carry out renewed filming of well-baby visits in cases that caused them concern, to assess their evolution and discuss new strategies within the interdisciplinary framework of the team.

Practitioners' experience with training and its integration into clinical practice

At the end of the second video filming of the infants, the practitioners were invited to a focus group (Silveira Donaduzzi et al., 2015; García Calvente and Mateo Rodríguez, 2000) to report on their experience with the training programme and its application in clinical practice. This meeting was coordinated by the author, and the following topics were discussed: the benefits or otherwise of training for clinical practice, the usefulness of the proposed approach and its benefits for the infant and its parents. **Table 10.2** presents illustrative quotations by category (Bonifacino, 2019).

Regarding the benefits of the training for the clinical practice, the practitioners mentioned that they felt better equipped for dealing with infants and their parents, being more aware of the dyad's emotional needs and more confident about their capacity to attend to and understand the infant's expressions and initiatives. They highlight that the training increased their ability to observe the infant and allowed them to pay more attention to and make sense of his/her reactions during the interaction. In addition, the practitioners reported that understanding the centrality of early interaction for the infants' present and future health and development fosters more active and spontaneous interaction with the infant, which was encouraged by the training.

As for the usefulness of the approach, the practitioners underlined that the training exploited the full potential of the well-baby visit for infant health care and pointed out the flexibility of the approach, its contribution to risk detection, and an educational value in providing a way of showing parents the communicational capacities of their children.

In relation to the benefits of this approach for infants and their parents, practitioners recognise an increase in the quality of care and make better use of time during the well-baby visit. They also noted an effect on mothers, observing that they were more involved, more attentive in subsequent consultations and more attentive to the infant's emotional expressions and aspects of the interaction, which they spontaneously discussed with the doctor. The practitioners also noted mothers' greater self-esteem in their maternal role, while they perceived more recognition and responsibility for themselves for their children's development.

Finally, the practitioners expressed the importance of this work not only for their regular clinical practice, but also for the functioning of the health centre itself, taking into account the adversity of the setting and the institutional difficulties. All of them agreed that the bi-weekly team meetings generated a motivating climate of participation and collaboration in the search for resources for the benefit of the infant. They also noted the importance of joint observation of video footage of well-baby visits and the expectation of sharing their concerns about the infants, as well as their satisfaction with

Table 10.2 Focus group data. Practitioners' experience in the training programme and its implementation in clinical practice.

Categories	Illustrative quotations
1. Benefit of the training for clinical practice	• "This training changed how the parents and we saw the infant and broadened our concept of the healthy infant." (1) • "It systematises the observation of the infant, and we can share it in the team meetings." (5) • "After the training, what we observe makes more sense, and we observe more details. Prior to this, I would observe something that seemed strange to me but I did not know why, and I immediately made a referral because I did not know what was happening with the infant nor what to do." (2) • "We are more active with the infant during the consultation, we interact more, we seek [more contact with] him/her. Before the training, I paid more attention to other things." (3) • "I always talked to the infant . . . Before the training, I did so intuitively . . . Now I know that this is good and that when the mother sees the infant interacting, she is discovering something new." (4)
2. Usefulness of the approach	• "This work generated a more acute valuation of the infant's development, and it is useful for all the disciplines." (6) • "This approach is useful not only for detection but also for strengthening the healthy infant's capacities, as well as showing the parents that a two months-old infant has many capacities for communication." (2) • "It allows us to benefit from existing resources in a better way. It is simple, it does not require extra time or equipment and we are used to using scales, it is common in medical language." (1) • "The approach is also useful for providing the mother with resources during the home visit." (7)
3. Benefits of the approach for the infant and his/her parents	• "This approach promoted a better appreciation of the infant's development by the parents." (5) • "It became a tool that had an impact on the mother. Indirectly, through a better appreciation of the infant, the mother felt herself to be more important and she felt more involved in the infant's health and development." (3) • "Infants' mothers were attentive in the subsequent consultation, and they encouraged a greater participation of the father." (7) • "Mothers gave more attention to aspects related to their infants' emotional development and interaction and were more stimulating with them." (4)

Note: Professional identification of participants: paediatricians (1–4), family doctor (5), child nutritionist (6), paediatric nurse (7).

the favourable evolution. At the same time, they recognised that the group learning and interdisciplinary dialogue in the fortnightly meetings gave them a sense of institutional identity and belonging. They added that the motivating atmosphere generated by this work transcended the team of participating practitioners, encouraging the voluntary collaboration of the assistant porters and nurses of the health centre in the filming of the consultations. Finally, they expressed their expectation to continue functioning as a team in implementing this approach and holding monthly meetings at the health centre, to which they would invite new practitioners, in order to reach more infants and their parents.

In summary, the practitioners' exchange during the focus group showed that they experienced the programme training as a positive contribution that broadened their perspective of infant health and well-being and changed their clinical practice by offering them new strategies for risk identification and for timely interventions to the benefit of the infant and her/his parents. Moreover, they reported that this work allowed them to measure the impact of the quality of paediatric follow-up care on the development and mental health of these highly socially vulnerable infants. This perception is confirmed by the quantitative results presented in the following chapter.

References

American Academy of Pediatrics. (2019). *Agenda for children: Medical home.* Washington, DC: AAP. https://www.aap.org/en-us/about-the-aap/aap-facts/AAP-Agenda-for-Children-Strategic-Plan/Pages/AAP-Agenda-for-Children-Strategic-Plan-Medical-Home.aspx (Consultation 10 April 2022).

Bonifacino, N. (2010). Jardín maternal. Un espacio para la promoción de salud [Daycare centre. A space for health promotion]. In G.Albónico (Ed.). *Otra voz en la Educación [Another voice in education]*. Montevideo: Ed. Psycholibros.

Bonifacino, N. (2019). *Programa de formación a profesionales de la salud en detección de retraimiento infantil y promoción de la interacción temprana durante la visita pediátrica* (doctoral thesis). University of Valencia, Spain. Doctoral Programme in Perinatal and Infant Psychology and Psychopathology. https//roderic.uv.es

Bonifacino, N., Lezama, G., Nauar, M., Llaguno, N. and Simó, S. (2023). Detección precoz de desviaciones y promoción de las habilidades sociales el lactante con la escala ADBB durante el seguimiento pediátrico. Experiencia en un centro de salud pública de alta vulnerabilidad social [Early detection of deviance and promotion of social skills in infants with the ADBB scale during paediatric follow-up. Experience in a public health centre of high social vulnerability]. *Archivos Pediatría de Uruguay, 94*(2), e218. https://doi.org/10.31134/AP.94.2.

Bonifacino, N., Musetti, D., Plevak, A. and Schelotto, M. (2011). La consultation en pédiatrie: la première approche à la santé mentale des enfants [The consultation in paediatrics: The first approach to children's mental health]. *Devenir, 23*(2), 117–127. https://doi.org/10.3917/dev.112.0117.

Bonifacino, N., Plevak, A., Musetti, D. and Silveira, A. (2014). Retraimiento sostenido: Un indicador de riesgo en el desarrollo temprano. Detección e intervención en el primer nivel con la escala ADBB [Sustained withdrawal: A risk indicator in early development. Detection and intervention at the first level with the ADBB scale. Experience in two public health centres in the metropolitan area]. *Archivos Pediatría de Uruguay, 85*(1), 30–38.

Boyce, W., Levitt, P., Martinez, F., McEwen, B. and Shonkoff, J. (2021). Genes, environments, and time: The biology of adversity and resilience. *Pediatrics, 147*(2), e20201651. https://doi.org/10.1542/peds.2020-1651.

Brazelton, T. (1994). Touchpoints: Opportunities for preventing problems in the parent-child relationship. *Acta Paediatrica, 394*, 35–39. https://doi.org/10.1111/j.1651-2227.1994.tb13212.x.

Carey, W. (2010). Coping with children's temperament. In M. Leuzinger, J. Canestry and M. Target (Eds.). *Early development and its disturbances.* London: Karnac.

Fonagy, P., Gergely, G., Jurist, E. and Target, M. (2002). *Affect regulation, mentalization, and the development of the self.* New York: Other Press.

Fox, S., Levitt, P. and Nelson, C. III. (2010). How the timing and quality of early experiences influence the development of brain architecture. *Child Development, 81*(1), 28–40. https://doi.org/10.1111/j.1467-8624.2009.01380.x.

García Calvente, M. and Mateo Rodríguez, I. (2000). El grupo focal como técnica de investigación cualitativa en salud: Diseño y puesta en práctica [The focus group as a qualitative health research technique: Design and implementation]. *Atención Primaria, 25*(3), 181–186.

Garner, A. and Yogman, M. (2021). Preventing childhood toxic stress: Partnering with families and communities to promote relational health. *Pediatrics, 148*(2), e2021052582. https://doi.org/10.1542/peds.2021-052582.

Leblanc, N. and Soulé, M. (1995). La información y capacitación del personal. [Staff information and training]. In S. Lebovici and F. Weil Halpern (Eds.). *La psicopatología del lactante [The psychopathology of the infant].* Buenos Aires: Siglo XXI.

Lebovici, S. and Weil-Harper, F. (1995). *La psicopatología del bebé [The psychopathology of the baby].* Siglo XXI.

Puura, K., Malek, E. and Berg, A. (2018). *Integrating infant mental health at primary health care level.* Tampere: World Association for Infant Mental Health. https://perspectives.waimh.org/2018/04/27/integrating-infant-mental-health-at-primary-health-care-level/ (Consultation 20 April 2022).

Shah, P., Muzik, M. and Rosenblum, K. (2011). Optimizing the early parent-child relationship: Windows of opportunity for parents and pediatricians. *Current Problems in Pediatric and Adolescent Health Care, 41*(7), 183–187. https://doi.org/10.1016/j.cppeds.2011.02.002.

Shonkoff, J., Boyce, W., Levitt, P., Martinez, F. and McEwen, B. (2021). Leveraging the biology of adversity and resilience to transform paediatric practice. *Pediatrics, 147*(2), e20193845. https://doi.org/10.1542/peds.2019-3845.

Silveira Donaduzzi, D., Colomé Beck, C., Heck Weiller, T., Nunes da Silva Fernandes, M. and Viero, V. (2015). Focus group and content analysis in qualitative research. *Index de Enfermería, 24*(1–2), 71–75.

Spitz, R. (1945). Hospitalism: An inquiry into the genesis of psychiatric conditions in early childhood. *Psychoanal Study Child, 1*, 53–74.

Stern, D. (1995). *The motherhood constellation: A unified view of parent-child psychotherapy.* Oxford: Routledge.

Tronick, E., Als, H., Adamson, L., Wise, S. and Brazelton, T. (1978). Infant response to entrapment between contradictory messages in face-to-face interaction. *Journal of the American Academy of Child and Adolescent Psychiatry, 17*(1), 1–13.

Winnicott, D. (1956 [1958]). Primary maternal preoccupation. In *Collected papers: Through paediatrics to psycho-analysis.* London: Tavistock, pp. 300–305.

Winnicott, D. (1960 [1981]). Theory of the parent-infant relationship. In *The maturational process [and the facilitating environment]* (Spanish ed.). Barcelona: Laia.

Worthman, C., Plotsky, P., Schechter, D. and Cummings, C. (Eds.). (2010). *Formative experiences: The interaction of caregiving, culture, and developmental psychobiology.* Cambridge: Cambridge University Press. https://doi.org/10.1017/CBO9780511711879.

11 Detection of withdrawal and promotion of early emotional development during the paediatric visit in a public health centre of high psychosocial risk in Uruguay[1]

1 1st Mention of the X Prize of Infant and Youth Mental Health Research organized by the Journal of child and adolescent psychopathology and mental health and supported by the city council of Saint Boi de Llobregat, Barcelona, Spain, (2023).

This chapter presents the effects of the training of primary care professionals in risk detection and the promotion of early emotional development on a group of infants at high psychosocial risk (Chapter 10) that are followed up in well-baby visits by practitioners who applied this knowledge in their clinical practice. The effect of this approach was assessed through the detection of withdrawal behaviour in these infants and in comparison with another group seen in the same health centre without the proposed approach.

This is action-based research work carried out with a quantitative methodology that enabled results with rigorous parameters shared by all disciplines to be obtained. This study was originally published in the official journal of the Sociedad de Pediatría of Uruguay with a systematic and detailed description of the method and data analysis (Bonifacino et al., 2023) and was published in the same format in the Revista de Psicopatología y Salud Mental del Niño y el Adolescente [Journal of child and adolescent psychopathology and mental health] published by the Orienta Foundation, Barcelona, Spain (Bonifacino et al., 2024). For our present purposes I shall present these aspects in a limited way, focusing on the results obtained for the benefit of the infants and their parents.

Procedure for assessing infant withdrawal behaviour

In this study, the ADBB scale was used to screen for withdrawal behaviour in 101 infants during well-baby visits to a public health centre in an area of high social vulnerability (Chapter 10). A proportion of these infants (43) underwent the usual well-baby visit and were videoed during just one well-baby visit, between the ages of eight and 11 months. The remaining (58) had a well-baby visit with the four paediatricians and the family doctor who implemented the training programme and participated in the bi-weekly team meetings for the

DOI: 10.4324/9781032614823-14

supervision of the approach (Chapter 10). These infants attended well-baby visits with these practitioners for at least six months and were videoed twice in total, once between the ages of 2 and 5 months and then again between the ages of 8 and 11 months. This methodology was implemented to determine the evolution of withdrawal over time in these infants who were attended in the manner of the proposed approach and to compare the presence of withdrawal between this group and infants attending the usual well-baby visits at the same health centre and at the same ages.

All infants were born full term and without perinatal pathology, and no multiple births were included. The study was conducted in the real setting of a well-baby visit at the health centre and was approved by the institutions involved and by the Research Ethics Committee of the Faculty of Psychology of the University of the Republic (Uruguay). The informed consent of the parents was requested, including permission to have their infant's well-baby visits videoed, depending on which group they were in. Data were also collected that could have an impact on the presentation of withdrawal behaviour.

Figure 11.1 presents the flow chart of the study, with details concerning the practitioners involved (Chapter 10) and the procedure for assessing infant withdrawal.

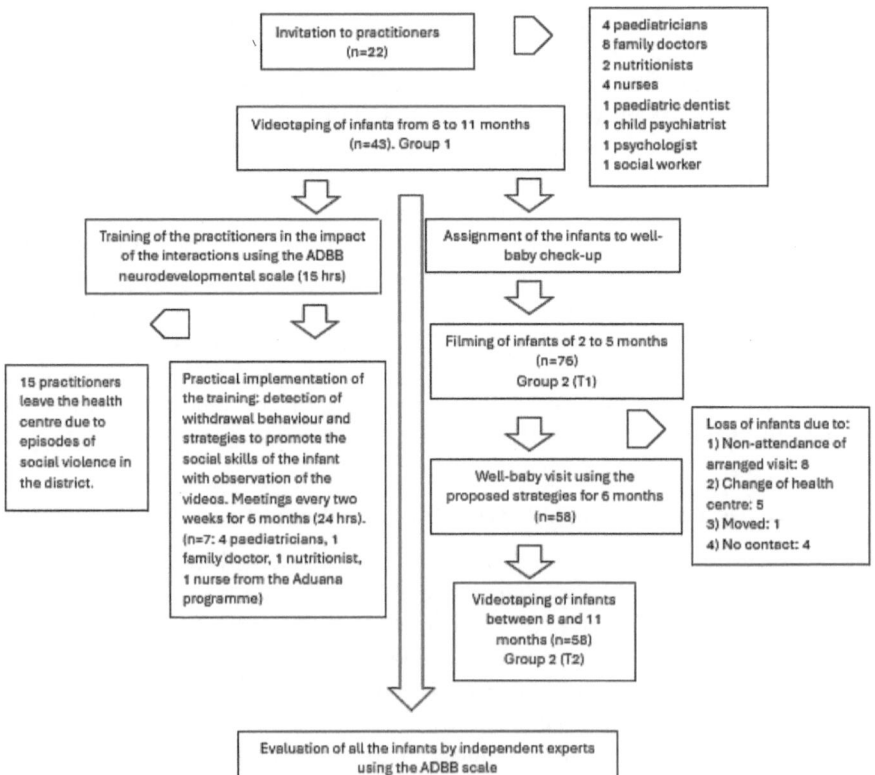

Figure 11.1 Flow chart of the study.

Video footage was taken of the corresponding well-baby visits, and the ADBB scale was used by at least two of three independent experts to assess all the infants as either exhibiting no withdrawal behaviour (ADBB score 0–4) or as withdrawn (ADBB score ≥ 5). These experts were three paediatricians from another public health centre who had previous training and experience with the ADBB scale and who received the video recordings randomly, unaware of any information about the infants or the group they came from.

Presence of withdrawal in infants and comparison between groups

Infant data and detection of withdrawal behaviour

Included in the statistical study were 43 infants who underwent the usual well-baby visits at the health centre and 58 who attended well-baby visits with the practitioners implementing the training programme and had a second filming at 8 to 11 months old. The analysis of socio-demographic characteristics between the two groups showed no statistically significant differences, allowing the comparison of withdrawal behaviour **(Table 11.1)**.

Table 11.1 Socio-demographic characteristics of both groups of infants (n = 101).

	Group assessed only once n = 43 n (%)	Group with two assessments n = 58 n (%)	Difference p
Infant characteristics			
Girls	22 (51)	24 (42)	0.219
Birth weight (grammes) Mean	3242 (SD = 529)	3373 (SD = 444)	0.133
Maternal characteristics			
Mean age (years)	25 (SD = 6.6)	24 (SD = 6.5)	0.605
Educational level			
Up to secondary education	24 (56)	36 (62)	0.182
Secondary education	19 (44)	22 (38)	
Paternal characteristics			
Mean age (years)	28 (SD = 7.5)	29 (SD = 8.3)	0.847
Educational level			
Up to secondary education	27 (63)	42 (72)	0.364
Secondary education	16 (37)	16 (28)	
Social characteristics			
Number of children in the household			
1 child	17 (40)	24 (41)	
1–3 children	17 (39)	23 (40)	0.806
>3 children	9 (21)	11 (19)	
Parental work status			
Unemployed	18 (44)	18 (33)	0.293
Working father	24 (56)	36 (67)	
Paternity			
Single mother	7 (16)	10 (18)	0.868
Mother and father cohabit	36 (84)	47 (82)	

Regarding the detection of withdrawal behaviour, in the application of the ADBB scale the experts detected 53% in the 43 infants seen in the regular paediatric visit, and the group in paediatric follow-up with the proposed approach presented 22% of withdrawal behaviour between 2 and 5 months of age and 14% between 8 and 11 months.

Comparison of the presence of withdrawal behaviour between groups

The group of infants in paediatric follow-up with the professionals applying the training programme showed no statistically significant differences in the presence of withdrawal between the two assessment periods **(Figure 11.2)**.

This result was contrary to our expectations. However, these results do show a clinical benefit, as several infants who were withdrawn at the first assessment are no longer withdrawn six months later.

Moreover, when this study was conducted in the real setting of clinical practice, several infants attended well-baby visits as newborns with the practitioners who were already applying their new strategies, while the first assessment using the ADBB was not carried out until the infants were 2 months old, as indicated by the validation of this tool. This situation may have contributed to the fact that the withdrawal of these infants between 2 and 5 months is significantly lower than that observed in a previous study with infants in a psychosocial risk context in Uruguay and similar age

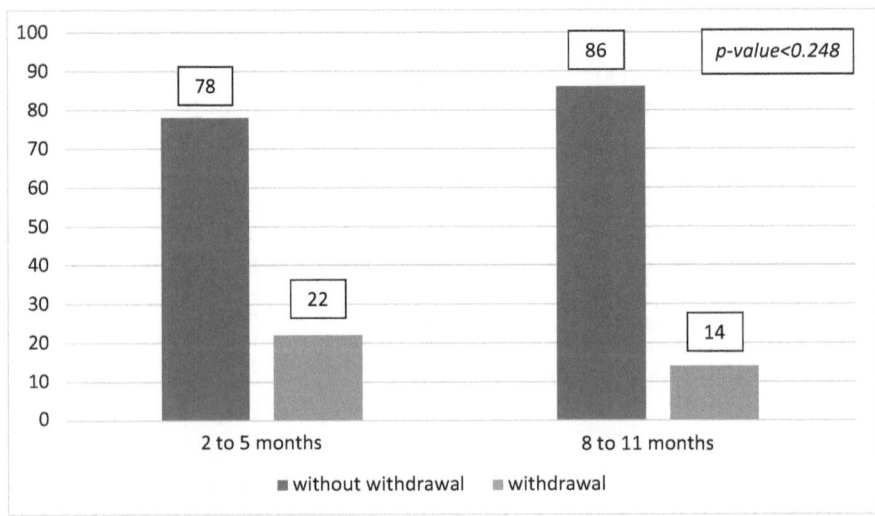

Figure 11.2 Percentage of withdrawal in the two evaluation periods of the group of infants attended by the professionals who implemented the proposed strategies (n = 58).

range (Bonifacino et al., 2014). In other words, the intervention of the practitioners before the first assessment may have had an effect.

Moreover, arguably the most relevant point in the results of this group is that withdrawal does not increase in the second assessment of this group, as would be expected in contexts of psychosocial risk and as was observed in a previous study of infants with routine well-baby visits (Bonifacino et al., 2014). In contrast, the withdrawal detected in the second assessment of these infants, between 8 and 11 months of age, is close to findings from international research conducted in contexts of lower psychosocial risk (Guedeney et al., 2013).

Finally, the comparison of the presence of withdrawal between both groups of infants between 8 and 11 months of age shows a statistically significant difference, which permits us to affirm that the infants attended with the proposed approach show less withdrawal behaviour than those who attended the usual well-baby visit **(Figure 11.3)**.

Given that none of the infants evaluated presented any organic pathology that would justify the presence of withdrawal behaviour, it is reasonable to suppose that the causes were relational and rooted in the parent-infant bond (Chapter 9). From this perspective, both the difference in withdrawal between the two groups between 8 and 11 months and the decrease in withdrawal behaviour in the second evaluation of the follow-up group using the proposed approach could be associated as an effect of the new resources implemented by the practitioners during the paediatric visits.

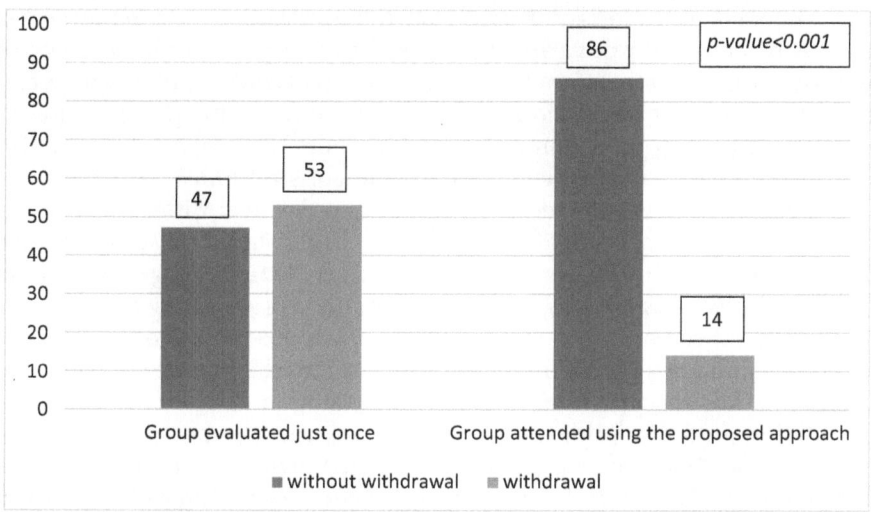

Figure 11.3 Percentage of withdrawal behaviour in both groups of infants between 8 and 11 months of age.

A hypothesis for the reduction of withdrawal behaviour in infants

The results show that the training had an impact on the practitioners' clinical practice, to the benefit of the infants. This situation leads to a reflection on the conditions that may have contributed to the reduction of withdrawal behaviour, even reversing the negative influence of the psychosocial risk context. In my view, these conditions involve different actors and correspond to different levels of experiences that are mutually interdependent in a complex interrelationship **(Table 11.2)**.

Firstly, as discussed in the previous chapter, the incorporation of training that allows the emotional needs of the mother-infant dyad and the importance of relational experiences for infant mental health to be taken into account promotes a change in the practitioner and their praxis (Chapter 10). This condition has implications for the infant and the mother or parents present at the well-baby visit.

With his or her new clinical positioning, the paediatrician or family doctor creates a favourable setting for the infant's resources to be deployed in communication and in the expression of his or her emotional experiences, thus placing the doctor-infant relationship at the centre of the well-baby visit. This context conveys to parents the practitioner's interest in and appreciation of the infant's communication skills, at the same time encouraging them to view their infant as having a psychic and an emotional life.

In this sense, although the training programme provides practitioners with a strategy guide that can favourably influence their communication with the infant (Chapter 10), these are presented by way of reference and are far from a protocolised intervention. That is to say, the change in the practitioner's attitude is not based on the application of a patterned or automatic behaviour but arises from his or her own sensitivity as a person and from his or her vocation for the service and care of infant health, which find new forms of expression according to the new knowledge acquired. According to the perception of the practitioners themselves (Chapter 10), these strategies reaffirm their own spontaneous attitudes, and the training gives them a greater sense of meaning and a new dimension. In this respect, one paediatrician affirms (Chapter 10): *"I always talked to the baby. I used to do so intuitively. Now I know that this is the right thing to do and that when the mother sees the baby interacting, she discovers something new."*

On the other hand, the incorporation of an observational tool for the early detection of signs of infant withdrawal into the practice of well-baby visits expands the practitioner's resources with an operational approach, facilitating interdisciplinary dialogue. From the perspective which we propose, the ADBB scale encourages the paediatrician or family doctor to observe the infant with the integration of two closely interrelated experiential registers. I am referring here to the overt behaviour of the infant's social skills and the expression of the emotional experiences underlying the doctor-patient interaction.

Table 11.2 Elements with an impact on the favourable evolution of infants in paediatric follow-up with practitioners who integrated the training into their clinical practice.

	Training in early emotional development	Training in the ADBB scale	Team meetings
Impact on the practitioner: **Recognition of the emotional needs of the dyad.**	• Knowledge about the emotional experience of the infant and the mother. • Change in the representation of the infant. • Ability to make sense of what is observed. • Increased confidence in practitioner resources for infant understanding and care.	• Systematisation of observation. • Detection of signs of developmental risk with an internationally validated instrument. • Increased observational acuity. • Facilitation of interdisciplinary dialogue based on observation of the infant with shared judgement.	• Practitioner exchanges on infant observation and development. • Coordination of actions for the benefit of the infant. • Framework of belonging, identity and practitioner motivation. • Reflective supervision.

⬇

Impact on clinical practice: **Change in the emotional experience of the practitioner, the infant and the mother.**	▶ The baby's behaviour is perceived as a source of information about an emotional state. ▶ Greater initiative, availability and commitment of the practitioner in relation to the infant. ▶ Mother/parent attention is directed towards the infant's communication skills and expression of emotions. ▶ Practitioner-mother therapeutic alliance with recognition of maternal expectations in the relationship with the doctor.

⬇

Impact on the mother: **New resources in the relationship with the infant.**	▶ Change in the infant's representation by integrating a psychic and emotional dimension. ▶ Discovery of the infant's new skills in communicating with the practitioner. ▶ Increased attention and relevance to aspects of interaction and emotional development. ▶ Appreciation of her own maternal capabilities and of herself in her maternal role.

Finally, a further element to highlight in this work was the functioning and cohesion of the team of participating practitioners, with the integration of different disciplines that provide care to infants and their parents at the health centre (paediatricians, family doctor, child nutritionist, paediatric nurse). This space generated a shared framework for training and interdisciplinary dialogue, which instilled a sense of motivation in the work and the pleasure of discovery in all its members, including the author. This context also allowed for reflective supervision of the approach, a condition that Leblanc and Soulé (1995) identify as relevant to sustaining the emotional dimension of the practitioner in the daily care of the infant and parents.

The doctor-infant encounter in the paediatric clinic

To conclude, I would like to share some segments of paediatric follow-up to illustrate the practitioner's already mentioned new positioning, with the implications it has for the dynamics of the well-baby visit and for the infant and its mother. The following account is based on the observation of video footage of some paediatric visits interspersed among others which were not videoed. Each of these films to which I will refer is approximately eight minutes long.

First videoed well-baby visit. Leo is 3 months old. Lying on his back on the gurney, he slowly moves his head from side to side with his gaze wandering, not settling on anything. His mother is standing next to him. She is a young woman, seemingly insecure and fearful. The paediatrician greets them and stands in front of the baby. Without taking her eyes off him, she talks to his mother, who tells her that Leo has been suffering from a cold and a cough.

The paediatrician turns to the baby, holds his head and speaks to him in a warm, high-pitched voice, trying to get his attention: *"Hello little one, how are you doing? What are you looking at over there? Were you interested in something there?"*

Leo keeps moving his head from side to side almost automatically, without fixing his gaze on anything. There is no change in his facial expression. Every now and then, he emits a brief, almost inaudible sound. The paediatrician notices this and, in an animated voice, says, *"You're making noises. Do you want to chat?"*

She waits a few moments. Receiving no response, she gently rests her open hand on the baby's belly and speaks to him again, slightly moving him. Leo continues to be unresponsive. He is noticeably disconnected from his surroundings. At a certain point, he stops moving his head. Noticing this, the paediatrician looks at him and speaks to him in a warm voice: *"Little one, what is it? What are you looking for over there?"* Leo resumes his head movements, gazing vaguely.

"Let's try it like this," the paediatrician says, gently tipping him upright, holding him by his back. Accompanying the movement with an animated voice, she says: *"Ooohhhhhhh . . . now you can look at us more comfortably."* She stands in front of Leo, seeking his gaze, and continues to speak to him in a warm voice. The baby does not look at her. Nor does he look at his mother. Then, telling him what she is going to do, the doctor places him face-down on the gurney. Leo makes slight efforts to raise his head, with partial success. *"Good! What a beautiful head, the way it goes along with the movement,"*

she says to the mother, showing her the baby's movement, adding, *"You saw that when I hold him, he also holds his head up. That's very good . . ."*

She then asks the mother about his vitamin intake and breast feeding while asking her to hold Leo in her arms for auscultation. In this new position, the baby continues his floating and uncertain head movements, with no change in facial expression and without seeking or responding to the gaze of the paediatrician or his mother. His little arms and legs hang loosely by his sides. The paediatrician then invites the mother to sit on a chair and hold Leo in her lap. *"That way you'll both be more comfortable,"* she says. She crouches down in front of the infant and listens to him again, holding his arm and talking to him in a warm voice. He shows no reaction and continues with his uncertain head movements. Crouching down to Leo's level, the doctor speaks to his mother in a soft, reassuring voice: *"Yes, he has a bit of a cold, but his lungs are fine."* At a certain point, the baby moves his arms and legs voluntarily for the first time. The paediatrician looks at him for a few moments under the mother's watchful eye, and then turns to him in a warm, encouraging voice: *"Ah! Now you're moving more. You liked sitting like that with Mummy."* The mother smiles shyly, while for the first time Leo briefly glances at the paediatrician. She looks back at him, speaking to him in a warm, slow voice: *"You are a beautiful little boy, but you have some mucus, and it makes you cough. And that bothers you, doesn't it?"* Leo smiles slightly, sits up a little and vocalises some small sounds. His mother, looking at him, gently shakes his leg, as if to stimulate him.

"Aha, now you want to look at me," says the paediatrician, in a soft and playful tone. *"What are you telling me? I think you were a bit serious before."* And turning to the mother, she adds in a different tone of voice, *"Or maybe he was a bit sleepy?"* She answers in the negative, while continuing to look at Leo and gently shaking his leg. Finally, the paediatrician gives the mother some instructions for Leo's cold and asks her to come back in a fortnight.

Comment: The paediatrician is very concerned about this infant. He has significant difficulties in establishing contact, and she uses a variety of resources to pursue the relationship while performing the routine paediatric check-up. She also notes the mother's fragility, speaking to her gently and in a reassuring tone and showing her some of the baby's skills, such as holding his head up.

Second video recording. At 5 months old, Leo's mother is sitting on a chair, and the boy is sitting on her lap. The paediatrician is talking to the mother and notices that the infant is looking at her. She stops what she is saying to look at him and speak to him in a warm, animated voice: *"Hello, little one, how are you?"* Leo holds her gaze for a few moments, his facial expression unchanged. *"Today you have to be a really good boy,"* she adds, looking at him and smiling. He averts his gaze, turning his head and arching his eyebrows slightly.

"Ah, you don't want to. You're not looking at me," says the paediatrician, feigning a certain disappointment. *"What's over there? There's something*

that's caught his eye, I think," she says to his mother, who looks where she is pointing. Then, she rests the stethoscope on Leo's chest. He looks at her, makes a few little sounds, and looks away again. She speaks to him again in a soft voice. He wobbles his head, turning it uncertainly from side to side, and when he meets the paediatrician's gaze, he pauses for a moment. She holds his arm and speaks to him softly, with an animated expression.

At a certain point, he takes the paediatrician's hand and slowly moves the stethoscope away from his chest. She helps him to hold it, while she looks at him and asks: *"What was it? Don't you like this?"* He looks intently at the stethoscope, while the paediatrician speaks softly to him. *"Ah, yes, you liked this."* He brings the stethoscope to his mouth, slowly. *"No! Not in your mouth, little one!"* says the paediatrician, in a laughing voice and looking at him. Leo looks at her for a moment. His attentive mother smiles shyly. The infant arches his eyebrows without much expression, and looks back at the paediatrician, who continues to auscultate him while speaking to him in a warm, animated voice every now and then. She also talks to his mother. She then goes behind the baby and rests the stethoscope on his back. Leo turns his head towards her but does not look her in the eye. *"Hello! You found me!"* she says. Leo turns around again. She returns to stand in front of him, at his height, and talks to his mother, while gently moving Leo's leg. Then she takes him by both hands and speaks to him in a warm voice, looking at him. He looks at her for a moment, averts his gaze, and then looks back at her every now and then. From this position, the paediatrician speaks to the mother: *"Did you see that he sometimes looks at me now? And at you, too. And that's very important!"*

Comment: Leo shows slight but significant changes. He is a little more reactive, achieves sporadic but brief eye contact and shows some moderate initiative. The paediatrician is still concerned about him. Based on a very acute observation capacity, she is very attentive to the baby's slight gestures, trying to give meaning and answers. Also, she encouragingly points out to his mother certain aspects that show an evolution.

From this point on, the well-baby visits continue monthly as usual, and sometimes more frequently because the mother is concerned about her child's cough or cold and requests an appointment. For the mother, the link with the paediatrician serves as a framework to contain her fears and anxieties about the infant's health. The vulnerability of the infant and also of the mother is thus presented in the paediatric visit.

Third video recording. Leo is 10 months old. He is sitting on his mother's lap and in front of the paediatrician's desk. He spontaneously picks up a toy, puts it in his mouth and looks at the paediatrician. She looks at him too, greets him in an animated way, and they both smile. In the meantime, in response to a question from the doctor, the mother says that Leo has a cough and a rattle in his chest. He stretches his arm in the direction of another toy on the desk and looks at the paediatrician. She gives it to him, and Leo puts it in his mouth. He smiles animatedly, looking at her and vocalising briefly. The paediatrician continues talking to the mother, while Leo picks up toys and puts them in his mouth one by one. The mother picks up some that fall on the floor. Leo sometimes looks at the paediatrician and says something. "*Ah, you liked that one,*" she says. And offering him another, she adds, "*And what about this one? Let's see?*" Leo takes it, vocalising in an animated and modulated way. He puts it in his mouth and looks at the paediatrician expectantly, raising and waving his arms in the air. She looks at him and smiles: "*What is it? What do you want to tell me today? What a little rascal you are!*" Leo replies, "*Ta! Ta!*", looking at her and smiling mischievously. The paediatrician laughs animatedly. She then asks his mother to carry him to the gurney while she moves the toys. Sitting with the toys in front of him, Leo looks at her, and in a playful tone she says, "*Hello!*" She repeats this in a cheerful, smiling voice. With the same attitude, he puts a toy in his mouth. "*Ah, you liked that one,*" she says. Leo looks at her and nods with an exaggerated, smiling gesture. "*Ah . . . ah . . .*" he exclaims. Then he looks at the stethoscope, which is on the gurney. He points to it and looks at the doctor.

"*What is it? Did you like this, too?*" she says, in an animated tone. Leo nods and makes happy, emphatic voices: "*Ah . . . ah . . .*" The paediatrician accompanies the baby's gestures with some of her own, accompanying them with her voice: "*Yes! Oh, yes, you are! You're a cheeky rascal! You like everything!*"

Then she auscultates him, and he protests with a frown, refusing. He picks up the stethoscope, looks at it and quickly tries to put it in his mouth. "*Noo, not in your mouth! Don't put that in your mouth,*" she says to him, in a warm and affectionately chiding voice, as she retrieves the stethoscope. Leo looks at her carefully and shows her a toy he is holding in his other hand. "*Ah, yes, you can put that in your mouth,*" she says, while continuing to auscultate him. The baby keeps picking up different toys, making animated vocal sounds and seeking the paediatrician's attention. She tells his mother that he is happy, fever-free and active and confirms that he has a bad cold, as his mother had noticed. Then, in a higher-pitched voice, she turns to Leo: "*Right, little one? You've got a cold, but what a good boy you've been today!*"

Leo looks at her and smiles, as he stretches his arm towards the doctor's face, looking at her. In a high-pitched, animated voice, and looking up at him with a smile, she says, "*What is it? I know. I know what you want! You are a rascal! You want my glasses. That's what you like! You're a cheeky rascal!*" Leo looks at her, laughs and nods vigorously. "*Ta . . . ta . . .*" he says. The paediatrician and the mother laugh at his cheekiness. She then turns to the mother: *You saw how cute he is. You saw how he looks at us and keeps looking at us now, you said that you had noticed it at home too.*" "*Yes, and now he plays with toys, and he is talking more,*" adds his mother.

Comment: Leo is evidently evolving well. His face is expressive, he seeks and sustains eye contact, vocalises in an animated way and displays initiatives that lead the paediatrician to enjoy the encounter. A fluid relationship is established in which both actively participate. Consistent with the clinical assessment, the use of the ADBB scale no longer detects signs of withdrawal. At the end of the consultation, the paediatrician shares with the mother her assessment of Leo's favourable evolution, and she intervenes in the relaxed and cheerful atmosphere of this meeting, expressing her own observations.

Fourth video recording. The well-baby visit I report on in the next section takes place when Leo is 24 months old. He is standing in the consulting room, holding onto his mother's leg. The paediatrician greets them and asks them how they have been. *"Good, he's talking now,"* says the mother, as she sits him on the gurney. The paediatrician approaches, and the toddler looks at her expectantly. *"What, darling, what's the matter?"* she asks him. He says something that is difficult to understand and reiterates it. *"Ah! You want a toy! Wait, I'll find one for you,"* she replies, reaching for a basket under the gurney. Leo follows her with his eyes, while his mother is taking off his clothes. *"He's taller, isn't he?"* comments the paediatrician. *"Yes, he's grown a lot,"* says his mother, with a smile.

The doctor gives Leo some toys: *"Here you are, here's a little colourful bucket, and I have a duck here, and there's a toy boat, too,"* she adds, looking at him and smiling.

He picks up the toys, looks at them, drops the duck and the toy boat into the bucket, making a noise, and looks at the paediatrician, saying something else. *"Yes. You played with the balls last time, but those are not there now,"* she says, looking at him. *"Ducky there,"* says Leo, pointing into the bucket and looking at the doctor. *"Yes, there's the ducky,"* she replies.

The paediatrician questions the mother about feeding and asks her to undress him. When she starts doing so, Leo says *"Noooo!"* with an exaggerated gesture of refusal and an angry expression. Then he looks at the paediatrician, again expectantly. *"Well, sweetie? And how do we get the ducky out now?"* she asks him. Leo, upturning the bucket with a smile, drops the duck so the paediatrician can see it. *"Oh, it's out!"* she says, looking at Leo with surprise. *"It's out!"* he reiterates, as the two look at each other and smile.

Leo continues to put toys in and take them out of the bucket and seeks to share this activity with the paediatrician, who responds with encouragement. While she is talking to his mother, Leo looks at her insistently, until, at a certain point, he interrupts the conversation and speaks to her, pointing his finger towards the basket of toys.

She looks at him. *"What else, darling?"* she asks him. Immediately, changing her tone of voice, the paediatrician turns to his mother: *"Wait a moment, because he wants something else. Let's see, what could it be?"*

"Do you want another toy?" she asks Leo. *"Yes,"* he replies, adding something else incomprehensible, while looking at the paediatrician expectantly.

"Is it something I lent you the other time?" she asks. Leo nods in affirmation and says, *"brum-brum."* *"The toy car! Ah! You want the toy car!"* she exclaims.

She asks his mother to please look in the toy basket and give it to him, while she continues his check-up.

Leo is pleased with the car his mother gives him. Then he struggles and protests insistently while the paediatrician tries to auscultate him. *"Let me listen to you a little while you play with the toy car,"* she says. But Leo insistently refuses, saying firmly *"No, no, no!"* and pushing the stethoscope away with his open hand, while holding the toy car in the other. *"I know you don't want to, how naughty you are,"* says the doctor, chiding him affectionately. *"Come on, Leo,"* adds his mother. He eventually allows himself to be examined under protest and giving his paediatrician a very serious look. When she finishes listening to him, he shows her that he has put the toys in the bucket again: *"Look! Gone in! Gone in!"* he says, getting her attention again.

Comment: Leo continued to progress favourably. His ability to relate and communicate now includes the incorporation of verbal language. He comes to the paediatric visit looking to reconnect. The relationship with the paediatrician is maintained, and the toddler comes with the confidence of feeling listened to and understood in his expectations, and she uses her interest, her memory and her sensitivity to accompany him in his experiences. From my point of view, this scenario, as well as the sequence presented in its entirety, highlights the fact that we should not underestimate the impact that the quality of the encounter with the practitioner in the setting of a well-baby visit can have for the infant and his mother, even during the limited time of each consultation.

Finally, it is necessary to recognise that neither the approach we propose nor the paediatric visit are always sufficient to promote a favourable evolution in the infant, and even less so considering the complexity of the psychosocial risk context and its consequences. However, in any case, and taking this reality into account, it is possible to consider that the different spaces of care for the infant and her parents are always an opportunity to approach and encounter the dyad, giving sensitive responses to the needs and experiences of both parties. From this perspective, this paper proposes that psychoanalytic tools can be transformed into useful and valuable resources to contribute to a culture of primary prevention and promotion of children's emotional development and mental health, with potential reach to different sectors of our society.

References

Bonifacino, N., Lezama, G., Nauar, M., Llaguno, N. and Simó, S. (2024). Detección precoz de desviaciones y promoción de las habilidades sociales el lactante con la escala ADBB durante el seguimiento pediátrico [Early detection of deviance and promotion of social skills in infants with the ADBB scale during paediatric follow-up]. Experiencia en un centro de salud pública de alta vulnerabilidad social [Early detection of deviance and promotion of social skills in infants with the ADBB scale during the well-baby visit. *Revista de Psicopatología y Salud Mental del Niño y el Adolescente [Journal of child and adolescent psychopathology and mental health]*, 43, 27–38.

Bonifacino, N., Lezama, G., Nauar, M., Llaguno, N. and Simó, S. (2023). Detección precoz de desviaciones y promoción de las habilidades sociales el lactante con la escala ADBB durante el seguimiento pediátrico [Early detection of deviance and promotion of social skills in infants with the ADBB scale during paediatric follow-up]. Experiencia en un centro de salud pública de alta vulnerabilidad social [Early detection of deviance and promotion of social skills in infants with the ADBB scale during the well-baby visit. Experience in a public health centre of high social vulnerability]. *Arch Pediatr Urug, 94*(2), e218. https://doi.org/10.31134/AP.94.2.

Bonifacino, N., Plevak, A., Musetti, D. and Silveira, A. (2014). Sustained withdrawal: An indicator of risk in early development. Detección e intervención en el primer nivel con la escala ADBB [Sustained withdrawal: A risk indicator in early development. Detection and intervention at the first level using the ADBB scale. Experience in two public health centres in the metropolitan area]. *Arch Pediatr Urug, 85*(1), 30–38.

Guedeney, A., Matthey, S. and Puura, K. (2013). Social withdrawal behaviour in infancy: A history of the concept and a review of published studies using the alarm distress baby scale. *Infant Ment Health Journal, 34*(6), 516–531. https://doi.org/10.1002/imhj.21412.

Leblanc, N. and Soulé, M. (1995). La información y capacitación del personal [Staff information and training]. In S. Lebovici and F. Weil Halpern (Eds.). *La psicopatología del lactante [The psychopathology of the infant]*. Buenos Aires: Siglo XXI.

Appendix

Early childhood education and care institutions as spaces for promoting early emotional development and child mental health

In this chapter, psychoanalytic tools are introduced into infant and young child care and educational facilities, providing resources for the protection of early emotional development and infant mental health.

These institutions face major challenges in their daily dynamics. The specific needs of early infancy in terms of healthy development are radically opposed to a collective care approach based on generalisable guidelines. How, then, can conditions be created that favour the subjectivation process in a collective care setting? And how can infant-parent bonding be fostered when the infant spends many hours a day at a day care facility?

I will put forward some reflections on this issue based on my experience derived from my role as the professional responsible for the mental health of a large number of infants and young children who attended an institution with this profile during their parents' working hours and on the bases of the works of reference authors.

Subjectivity in the collective care space

These lines assume that the necessary conditions for early emotional development and the process of subjectivation arise within the framework of a close affective bond between the infant and the caregiver (Chapter 2, Chapter 8). In this regard, Brazelton and Greenspan (2000) note that the first three years of life are critical for the development of intellectual capacities and the quality of relationships that the infant may establish in the future. The prerequisite for such development is the opportunity to establish an intimate, loving and stable bond with parents and a few caring adults.

As discussed in previous chapters, this perspective continues to be confirmed by the latest research (Chapter 8, Chapter 9). Given its importance for early development, this could be the starting point of any institution that receives infants and young children for their daily care. In other words, it is crucial to make this perspective a central axis of institutional life, thus encouraging an ongoing search for strategies which foster and preserve the conditions necessary for each infant's unique emotional development, even in the setting of collective care.

The first adjustment to be made in such organisations would be to ensure that the same caregiver welcomes the infant every day and takes care of him or her for most of the time. The physical proximity of the caregiver assuming a maternal role, together with his or her emotional availability and interest in relating, contribute to generate a certain empathy and identification with the infant's needs, promoting sensitive responses and initiatives (Winnicott, 1960, chap. 2).

In an organisation dedicated to infant development and mental health, it is essential to encourage this bond and affective proximity between the infant and the caregiver as a reference person. The infant or toddler must be able to identify the caregiver in the group setting, to seek and find the caregiver's gaze in order to understand his or her own emotional experiences, and to explore and discover the world creatively (Emde, 1998; Tomasello, 1999 and Tomasello and Haberl, 2003, cited by Fonagy and Target, 2007). Thus, even in the setting of an educational and early childhood care facility, it is important not to underestimate the influence of environmental provision at this sensitive and vulnerable stage in the individual's emotional development (Winnicott, 1957).

From this perspective, the day care centre radically distances itself from the concept of an extended pre-school environment with group offerings aimed in advance at providing systematic stimuli or cognitive development. Instead, it prioritises the emotional availability and adaptability of the caregiver in a relationship in which the infant perceives itself as having an active part. Early infant care facilities thus take on an identity of their own that transcends exclusively educational aspects. They essentially become interdisciplinary settings, in which educational objectives and the care of infant's development and mental health converge.

The parent-infant bond in day care facilities

The scenario outlined previously gives rise to a complex institutional dynamic, in which emotional experiences flow that involve all participants, especially infants, their parents and those on the front line of daily care (Bonifacino, 2010). In my experience, in this context the opening of regular spaces for interdisciplinary dialogue within the facility setting enables the relationship between the infant and the caregiver to be considered a subject for analysis and shared reflection. This teamwork, involving those on the front line of care, managers and physical and mental health practitioners engaged in the day-to-day activities of the facility, allows constant revision of institutional criteria and the positioning of each of those involved in the task. Moreover, in these dialogue spaces the caregiver's observation of the infant allows possible misunderstandings in the relationship to be identified, as well as the infant's own difficulties (Chapter 9). This scenario leads to the creation of new institutional resources, involving both day-to-day care and possible interventions with parents by physical and/or mental health professionals (Bonifacino, 2010).

In my experience, maintaining these regular spaces for interdisciplinary dialogue in the institutional dynamic reaffirms the commitment of all those involved in the task from their different functions, while at the same time expanding the resources of those on the front line of care, encouraging them to be flexible and sensitive to the infant and its parents. The following is a brief account of a situation that occurs daily in a day care centre, and which unexpectedly tests the caregiver's resources. It concerns a baby who, from the age of 2 months, spends eight hours a day – her parents' working hours – in a communal room in a day care facility. The situation presented here occurs at the end of the day.

The mother goes to the day care room where her 4-month-old daughter is. As she approaches, she hears the infant's gurgles and the caregiver's playful voice, softly and warmly mentioning the baby's name. She stops at the door and silently watches through the window. She quietly watches for a few moments as the caregiver and her daughter interact, look at each other and smile. Suddenly opening the door she speaks, her tone of voice lying somewhere between relief and regret: "Oh! Bea, the way she laughs with you!" Surprised that the mother is in the room, the caregiver turns the chair slightly so that the baby is facing her mother. Then, in an open and energetic tone, she says, "Look who's here, Annie! Oh good! Mummy's here!" The baby looks up and meets her mother's gaze, smiles at her and shows her excitement by vigorously moving her arms and legs. The relieved mother comes over, picks her up and hugs her warmly. The caregiver will later tell her how the baby spent the day.

In the context of the mother's own emotional sensitivity at this stage of her life, the figure of the caregiver providing for the infant's daily needs at the facility occupies a very significant place for her, one which is imbued with a certain ambivalence (Stern, 1995). On the other hand, the practitioner administering care from the perspective we propose is inevitably involved and emotionally invested in the relationship with the infant and its parents (Chapter 11). Her daily responses and attitudes can either evoke feelings of helplessness and frustration in the mother, or they can foster the encounter with her daughter, maintaining and recognising her role as a mother, as I have attempted to illustrate in the scene described previously. This subtlety and flexibility in the caregiver's response can only occur when s/he has clearly identified and internalised the institution's objectives, her own task and her professional stance towards the infant and its parents (Bonifacino, 2010, 2014).

This scenario is built on the basis of institutional functioning that takes the infant's daily relationship with its caregiver as a subject for reflection and sustained analysis, within an interdisciplinary framework. This perspective prioritises the role of those who are in the first line of care at nurseries, positioning these practitioners in their daily work as agents of care and encouragement of the parent-infant bond and infant emotional development.

References

Bonifacino, N. (2010). Jardín maternal y promoción de salud mental [Daycare facilities and mental health promotion]. In G. Albónico (Ed.). *Otra voz en la educación [Another voice in education]*. Montevideo: Psicolibros Waslala.

Bonifacino, N. (2014). *Los primeros años de vida: etapa clave en el desarrollo del sujeto [The first years of life: A key stage in the development of the subject]*. Training Centre of the Uruguayan Institute for Children and Adolescents (CENFORES). Presidency of the Republic. www.inau.gub.uy

Brazelton, T. and Greenspan, S. (2000). *The irreducible needs of children*. Cambridge: Persus.

Emde, R. (1998). Yendo hacia adelante: Las influencias integradoras de los procesos afectivos en el desarrollo y en el psicoanálisis [Going forward: The integrative influences of affective processes in development and psychoanalysis]. *Psicoanálisis APdeBA, 20*(3), 473–516.

Fonagy, P. and Target, M. (2007). Playing with reality: IV. A theory of external reality rooted in intersubjectivity. *International Journal of Psychoanalysis, 88*, 917–937. https://doi.org/10.1516/ijpa.2007.917.

Stern, D. (1995). *The motherhood constellation: A unified view of parent-child psychotherapy*. Oxford: Routledge.

Tomasello M. (1999). *The cultural origins of human cognition*. Cambridge, MA: Harvard University Press.

Tomasello, M. and Haberl, K. (2003). Understanding attention: 12- and 18-month-olds know what is new for other persons. *Developmental Psychology, 39*, 906–912. 10.1037/0012-1649.39.5.906.

Winnicott, D. (1957 [1965]). On the contribution of direct child observation to psycho-analysis. In *The maturational process and the facilitating environment: Studies in the theory of emotional development* (Vol. 64). pp. 109–114. Barcelona: Laia

Winnicott, D. (1960 [1981]). Ego distortion in terms of true and false self. In *The maturational process* (Spanish ed.). Barcelona: Laia, pp. 169–184.

Index